Atlas of Arthroscopic Techniques

Atlas of Arthroscopic Techniques

William R Beach, MD
Tuckahoe Orthopaedics
Richmond, Virginia,
USA

T Duncan Tennent, FRCS, FRCS (Orth)
Department of Orthopaedic Surgery
St George's Hospital and Medical School
London,
UK

With contributions from

John F Meyers, MD
Terry L Whipple, MD
Richard B Caspari
Tuckahoe Orthopaedics
Richmond, Virginia,
USA

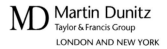
Martin Dunitz
Taylor & Francis Group
LONDON AND NEW YORK

First published in the United Kingdom in 2003
by Martin Dunitz Ltd, 11 New Fetter Lane, London EC4P 4EE

Tel.: +44(0) 20 7583 9855
Fax.: +44(0) 20 7842 2298
E-mail: info@dunitz.co.uk
Website: http://www.dunitz.co.uk

Although every effort has been made to ensure that all owners of copyright material have been acknowledged in this publication, we would be glad to acknowledge in subsequent reprints or editions any omissions brought to our attention.

Although every effort has been made to ensure that drug doses and other information are presented accurately in this publication, the ultimate responsibility rests with the prescribing physician. Neither the publishers nor the authors can be held responsible for errors or for any consequences arising from the use of information contained herein. For detailed prescribing information or instructions on the use of any product or procedure discussed herein, please consult the prescribing information or instructional material issued by the manufacturer.

A CIP record for this book is available from the British Library.

ISBN 1–85317–211–1

Distributed in the USA by:
Fulfilment Center
Taylor & Francis
10650 Toebben Drive
Independence, KY 41051, USA
Toll Free Tel.:   +1 800 634 7064
E-mail: taylorandfrancis@thomsonlearning.com

Distributed in Canada by:
Taylor & Francis
74 Rolark Drive
Scarborough, Ontario M1R 4G2, Canada
Toll Free Tel.: +1 877 226 2237
E-mail: tal_fran@istar.ca

Distributed in the rest of the world by:
Thomson Publishing Services
Cheriton House
North Way
Andover, Hampshire SP10 5BE, UK
Tel.: +44 (0)1264 332424
E-mail: salesorder.tandf@thomsonpublishingservices.co.uk

Composition by J&L Composition, Filey, North Yorkshire, UK
Printed and bound in Spain by Grafos S.A. Arte Sobre Papel

CONTENTS

FOREWORD

Since the early era of arthroscopy much has evolved regarding the ease of performing arthroscopic surgery. We have progressed to a point where arthroscopy is clearly the treatment of choice for many procedures, and these procedures themselves are becoming more complex. By producing this book the authors have aimed to provide visual reinforcement of the experience gained in the operating room and to prepare the junior surgeon for safe and competent arthroscopic surgery. Tuckahoe Orthopaedics and Orthopaedic Research of Virginia, under the guidance of Drs Meyers, Whipple and the late Dr Caspari, have been instrumental in developing arthroscopic procedures over the last 20 years. We have included these as well as others which are reproducible and beneficial for our patients, and we would like to share these with other arthroscopists of all skill levels. We certainly do not suggest that our way of performing arthroscopic surgery is the only way. The use of a variety of instruments and implants is illustrated in the chapters that follow. The field of arthroscopy is developing so rapidly that the reader should not assume that the authors endorse any particular device, or that it is necessarily the 'best'. Some are used because we are comfortable with them even though they may not be state of the art. What is important throughout the text is the principle of the technique. The fine details should be adapted to suit local circumstances and preferences. Likewise, we have not described details of post-operative management and leave this to the personal preference of the individual surgeon.

No book can hope to be all things to all readers. The aim of this book is not to replace teaching in the operating rooms, but to supplement teaching and reading with images from real cases.

The early sections of each chapter on preparation and draping of the patient will not be relevant to the more experienced surgeon, and conversely the sections on ligament reconstruction and rotator cuff repair will be beyond the novice.

We hope that the techniques we describe, with the additional 'tips' to assist with the procedure, will be of as much benefit to other surgeons as they have been to us at Tuckahoe Orthopaedics.

A great debt is owed to the contributors to this book, without whom it would not have been possible. Both of the authors have been fellows at Orthopaedic Research of Virginia. Dr Caspari continued to teach regularly until his untimely death, and his legacy persists as a result of the techniques he developed and his enthusiasm for innovation and teaching. Dr Whipple also continues to have a great influence on the teaching of the fellows, both with the techniques he has pioneered and with his superb clinical teaching. Current fellows are fortunate to still benefit from Dr Meyers' arthroscopic knowledge and experience and a constant desire to take arthroscopy further forward. Without these surgeons, innovators and teachers this book would not have been possible and we are grateful.

We have greatly benefited from our mentors' commitment and dedication to education. The greatest gift is the gift of knowledge and the greatest testimony is the patience and friendship of a teacher. We are therefore ever indebted to these three pioneers and educators. We hope you can also benefit from their teaching through this arthroscopic atlas.

WRB
TDT

1 KNEE ARTHROSCOPY

INTRODUCTION

The knee was the first joint to be arthroscoped, and for nearly all surgeons is the joint in which they obtain their first experience of arthroscopic procedures. In this chapter we describe and illustrate a number of aspects of knee arthroscopy, from patient setup to anterior cruciate ligament (ACL) reconstruction.

There are many ways of doing all of the things described in this chapter and we do not claim that ours is the only way. We have, however, found that the techniques described here are reproducible, safe, and facilitate good arthroscopic surgery. Not everyone will want to use a leg holder; however, all surgeons should perform an examination under anaesthetic prior to arthroscopy. Likewise, although many surgeons will not use the Endobutton to secure the femoral side of an ACL graft, we have found it to be quick, easy and reliable. The principles of tibial and femoral tunnel placement and adequate notchplasty will remain the same regardless of the fixation technique used.

Our hope is that surgeons reading this chapter will combine the information we present with their own experience and preferences. Only this way will arthroscopy progress and develop.

There are risks and complications associated with any surgical procedure and the surgeon must be familiar with these before attempting any procedure. The more common or serious ones are outlined here, but there are others which are less common. The surgeon must have knowledge of the applied anatomy of the region if damage is to be avoided.

Neurovascular risks

The anteromedial and anterolateral portals both risk damaging the infrapatellar branches of the saphenous nerve, from which painful neuromas can result. Likewise, the tibial incision for hamstring harvesting and ACL graft insertion can damage the same nerves. This incision also risks damaging the main saphenous nerve as it continues down the medial aspect of the leg.

The same nerve is also at risk during placement of the posteromedial portal and the incision for plication of the vastus medialis obliquus. Likewise, the nerve may be damaged during repair of the medial meniscus when using the inside-out technique, and care must be taken to blunt dissect down to the capsule before tying down the sutures.

The common peroneal nerve lies in close proximity to the posterolateral portal and may be caught in sutures placed during repair of the lateral meniscus if the same meticulous attention to detail is not observed. Dissection prior to suture passage and the use of a protective guide help with this.

The tibial artery lies in close proximity to the posterior capsule and is placed at risk when instruments are used in this region. This is of particular concern during ACL surgery and if attempting to repair the posterior horn of either meniscus using the inside-out technique. Concern for the artery usually limits the extent to which the procedure can be used.

Complications

Infection is fortunately a very rare occurrence following knee arthroscopy, but meticulous care must still be taken at all stages. Some surgeons routinely give antibiotics prior to surgery, and this should certainly be considered if any material is to be inserted into the joint (meniscal repair, ACL reconstruction etc.).

Inside the joint itself the most common complication is chondral damage. This usually occurs as a result of poor instrument control and the shaver is the usual offender. Care must be taken when introducing or removing any instrument into the joint. Always watch the instrument enter and leave the joint. If using a shaver, turn the instrument so that the cutting surface is inferior. This will reduce the risk of gouging the femoral condyle should the instrument slip. If difficulty is encountered passing the instruments into the joint, or from one compartment to another, use the blunt trocar and sheath to create the passage. Remove the trocar and use the sheath to guide the instrument.

Meniscal damage is less common, but can occur if the medial portal is not made under direct vision. It is possible to pass the knife under, or through, the meniscus. By using the spinal needle to locate the correct position for the portal placement and watching the knife blade as it enters the joint, this complication can be avoided.

SETUP FOR KNEE ARTHROSCOPY

Most surgeons obtain their first exposure to arthroscopy with the knee. Knee arthroscopy is simpler than that of the other joints but still requires meticulous attention to all aspects of the surgery, including patient preparation. The authors prefer to arthroscope the knee with the thigh in a leg holder and the foot of the table lowered. This provides good access to all aspects of the joint and does not require a different setup for different procedures. This is especially useful if intraoperative findings necessitate a different procedure from that which was previously planned. Whatever the setup used, it is the responsibility of the operating surgeon to ensure that the patient is appropriately placed on the operating table so that full access is available. For example, when the foot of the table is lowered it will be possible to flex and extend the knee fully. Once the leg has been prepared and draped it is too late to move it. Likewise, ensure that the tourniquet is as high as possible and appropriately padded, and that the leg holder lies over the tourniquet and is secure. If it is at all possible that a posteromedial portal may be made, ensure that the contralateral leg is abducted as far as possible to facilitate access.

These are all simple steps, but ones which can easily be forgotten by both junior and experienced surgeons alike.

The patient is brought to the operating room and placed in the supine position on the operating table. Patients routinely undergo general anaesthesia.

A tourniquet is applied one to two handbreadths above the superior pole of the patella. Whether or not it is inflated is the preference of the surgeon, but applying it at this time is much better than trying to apply it later in the procedure (Fig. 1.1).

Much information may be ascertained from the examination under anaesthesia. A Lachman's test is demonstrated to check the competency of the anterior cruciate ligament (ACL). At 20–30º of knee flexion an anterior stress is placed on the tibia while the femur is stabilized (Fig. 1.2). An anterior drawer test is performed at 90º to further evaluate the ACL.

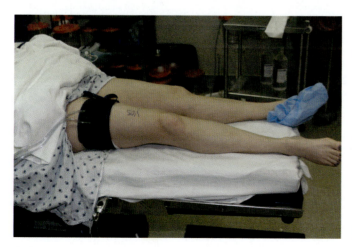

1.1

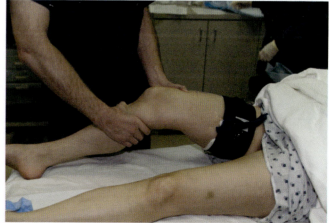

1.2

Another valuable test of the ACL is the pivot shift manoeuvre. While internally rotating the tibia with a valgus stress the knee is flexed and extended gently. Any significant gliding or subluxation of the tibia on the femur is indicative of an ACL injury (Fig. 1.3).

Varus and valgus stress tests are performed to test the competence of the medial collateral ligament (MCL) and the lateral collateral ligament (LCL) (Fig. 1.4).

Prior to elevation of the tourniquet an esmark bandage is applied. The knee is maximally flexed and the tourniquet inflated to 350 mm of pressure for the normal-size leg (Fig. 1.5). Very large legs will sometime require pressures of 400 mm, with a longer and wider cuff.

A knee holder is routinely used to stabilize the leg. This type of holder allows both varus and valgus stresses to be applied and is extremely stable because it attaches on both sides of the operating table (Fig. 1.6).

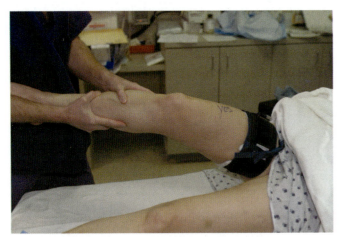

1.3

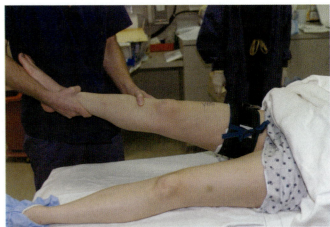

1.4

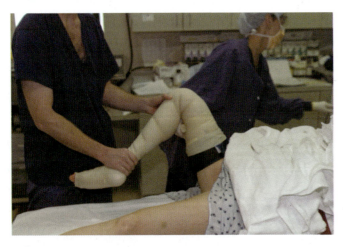

1.5

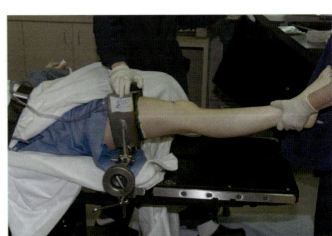

1.6

The knee holder is tightened around the tourniquet and the lower section of the bed is flexed out of the way (Fig. 1.7).

The contralateral lower extremity must be padded.

A betadine preparation is then applied to the leg from the tourniquet to the ankle (Fig. 1.8).

Draping begins with a plastic 'U' drape with adhesive tails (Fig. 1.9).

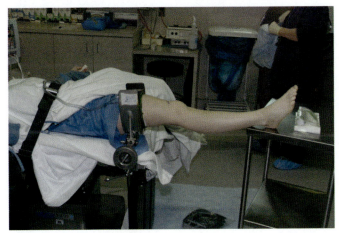

1.7

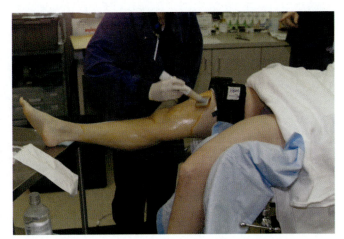

1.8

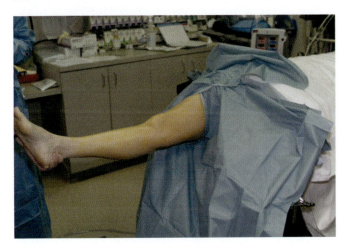

1.9

A sterile stockinette is then placed over the foot and tightly coapted to the foot and calf with a sterile bandage. The bandage should extend above the stockinette to prevent the arthroscopic fluid from flowing into the impervious stockinette, down to the non-sterile foot and then moving back out (Fig. 1.10).

The last drape is the extremity drape with a rubber dam. This slides up to the 'U' drape and forms the sterile barrier (Fig. 1.11).

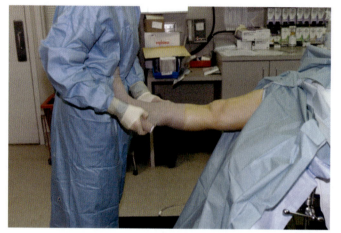 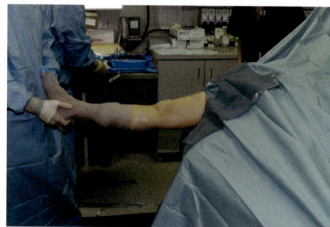

1.10   1.11

BILATERAL KNEE SETUP

Occasionally the need arises to arthroscope both knees. Setup and draping are the same as for a single leg, with few exceptions. The patient begins in the supine position and undergoes induction of anaesthesia. Both tourniquets are applied at this time (Fig. 1.12).

The leg holder is in position and the leg to be operated on first is exsanguinated and this tourniquet is inflated (Fig. 1.13).

A 'U' drape is carefully applied to one leg, so as not to contaminate either knee (Fig. 1.14).

The second 'U' drape is applied to the other knee (Fig. 1.15).

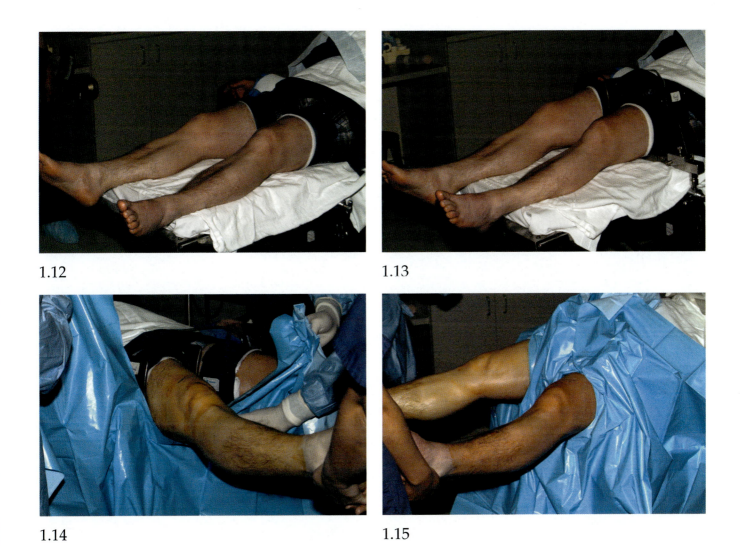

1.12

1.13

1.14

1.15

Both stockinettes are placed on the legs and wrapped with a sterile bandage (Fig. 1.16).

A bilateral extremity drape with a double fenestrated rubber dam fits over the feet and is slid up to the 'U' drapes.

To insure the sterility of the second operative leg another stockinette is placed over the first. The arthroscopy proceeds as a single knee scope (Fig. 1.17).

At the conclusion of the first procedure 30 ml marcaine and adrenaline are injected into the portal sites and the joint (Fig. 1.18).

A sterile dressing is applied to the first knee and the tourniquet is released. The stockinette is removed from the second leg and the leg exsanguinated with a sterile esmark. The tourniquet is inflated and the procedure is begun (Fig. 1.19).

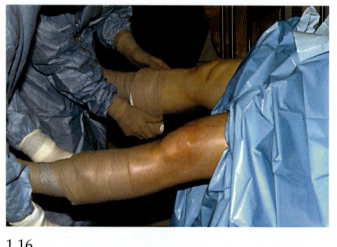

1.16

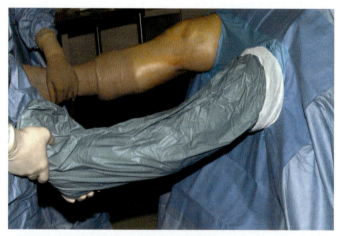

1.17

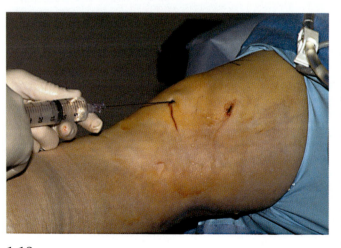

1.18

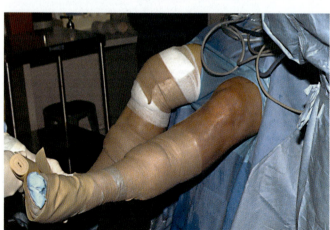

1.19

PORTAL CREATION

Creation of the portals is the most basic component of knee arthroscopy, but if proper care and consideration is not exercised it can make the procedure significantly more difficult and result in unwanted complications.

The anterolateral portal is always made blind, and it is important that the knife is advanced slowly into the soft spot. This particularly applies to both the very obese, when the landmarks may be difficult to identify reliably, and the very thin, where there is little subcutaneous tissue and it is theoretically possible to inflict femoral condyle damage.

Creation of the anteromedial portal risks damaging the medial meniscus and the infrapatellar branch of the saphenous nerve. Also, creation in the wrong place makes subsequent joint access difficult and may preclude surgery on the more posterior aspects of the joint. Although little can be done to prevent nerve damage (except for the possibility of using a transverse rather than a vertical skin incision), simple steps will eliminate the risk of meniscal laceration. These are detailed in the chapter but basically involve using a spinal needle to plan the incision site and watching the blade as it enters the joint. This also eliminates the risk of chondral damage at the same time.

The posteromedial and posterolateral portals both risk neurological damage, and again both should be made under direct vision and a trocar should be used to push the nerve to one side if it is close.

The knee is prepared and draped in the standard fashion, with the tourniquet inflated after the leg has been exsanguinated.

For the majority of arthroscopic procedures gravity fluid inflow is all that is required with a single portal arthroscopic cannula. If significant bleeding is anticipated, e.g. during an anterior cruciate ligament reconstruction, a fluid pump is recommended.

The lateral parapatellar or anterolateral portal is the 'main' portal. This is located in the superior portion of a triangle created between the patellar tendon/patella, the lateral femoral condyle and the lateral tibial plateau. The tendency is to make this portal too low. Stay high in this triangle for the best vantage point (Fig. 1.20).

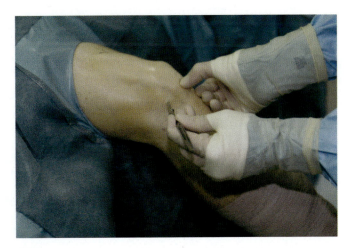

1.20

The direction of the portal incision is according to the surgeon's preference. A transverse incision starting at the patella/patellar tendon and extending laterally 4–5 mm reduces the risk of a neuroma of the infrapatellar branch of the saphenous nerve.

The anteromedial portal is the standard working portal and is made after the arthroscope has been introduced and the joint inspected. It is located medial to the patellar tendon and is usually lower than the lateral portal. An 18 g spinal needle is used to identify the correct position of the portal (Fig. 1.21).

The needle should lie above the meniscus and reach the region of the knee requiring attention (Fig. 1.22).

A small transverse incision is made through the skin and capsule under direct vision. If this is made 'blind' there is a risk of cutting the articular cartilage overlying the medial femoral condyle or the meniscus (Fig. 1.23).

A blunt trocar is pushed through the capsule to enlarge the capsular incision and facilitate instrument passage (Fig. 1.24).

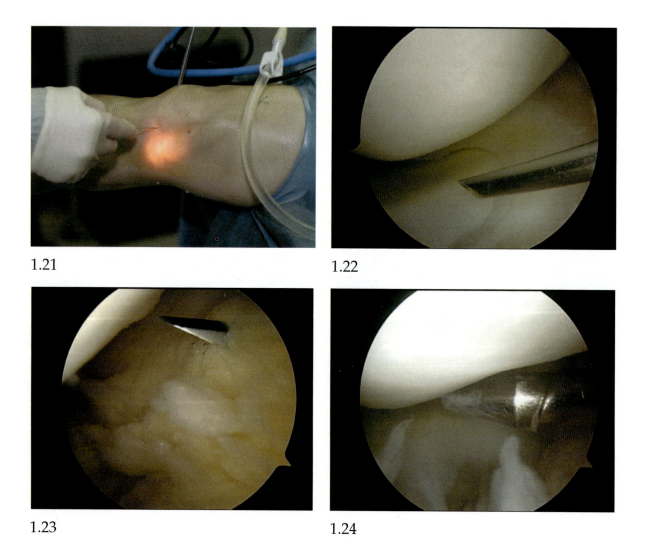

1.21

1.22

1.23

1.24

To facilitate the exchange of instruments through the anteromedial portal during the procedure the sleeve of the trocar can be left in situ. This will limit the size of the instruments that can be passed through, but does allow blood and debris to flow out of the knee (Fig. 1.25).

The posteromedial portal is used less frequently and mainly for accessing the back of the medial meniscus or a Baker's cyst.

The arthroscope is placed in the anteromedial portal and positioned against the lateral aspect of the medial femoral condyle. The blunt trocar is reinserted and the arthroscope driven through the intercondylar notch into the posterior compartment of the knee. A loss of resistance will be felt as the compartment is reached and the trocar will be held firmly in position if it is released from your hand (Fig. 1.26).

Alternatively, this may be done under direct vision in some cases. Position the arthroscope over the medial tibial spine and 'aim' at the space lateral to the lateral wall of the medial femoral condyle (Fig. 1.27).

By gently rotating the light source as the arthroscope is advanced the arthroscope can be steered into the posteromedial compartment (Fig. 1.28).

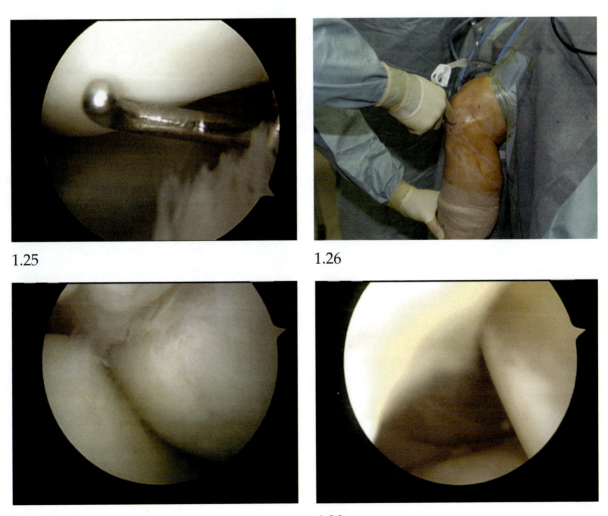

1.25

1.26

1.27

1.28

Once the arthroscope is in the posterior compartment rotate the light source so that the posterior aspect of the medial femoral condyle and the posteromedial capsule can be seen (Fig. 1.29).

Indent the posteromedial capsule with a finger to guide portal placement (Fig. 1.30).

If this is not possible (due to obesity) turn down the operating room lights. The arthroscope will transilluminate the skin, guiding the portal placement. This may also reveal the saphenous vein and nerve, reducing the chance of damaging them (Fig. 1.31).

As with the anteromedial portal, use an 18 g spinal needle to locate the correct site for the portal (Fig. 1.32).

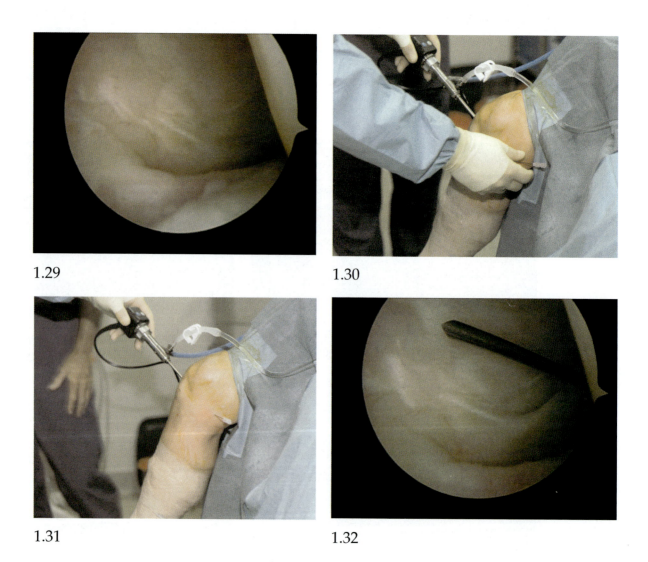

1.29

1.30

1.31

1.32

Once the position has been confirmed, make a small incision through the skin only to reduce the chance of neurovascular damage (Fig. 1.33).

Use the sharp trocar and cannula to push through the capsule under direct vision (Fig. 1.34).

Once the cannula is in the joint the trocar can be removed and instruments introduced (Fig. 1.35).

The posterolateral portal is made in the same manner as the posteromedial, taking care to avoid damage to the common peroneal nerve (Fig. 1.36).

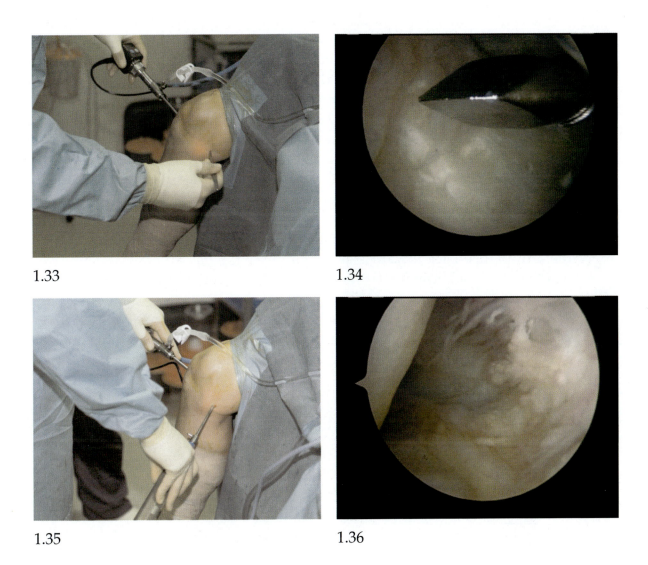

1.33

1.34

1.35

1.36

NORMAL KNEE ARTHROSCOPY

Careful history taking, examination and the appropriate use of preoperative investigations should make the 'normal knee arthroscopy' something that is never seen. Indeed, the images used to illustrate this chapter have been taken from several arthroscopic examinations in which a part of the knee was normal. This chapter is included because it is essential that the normal anatomy is appreciated, and a systematic routine must be followed for all examinations. Only in this way will the examination be complete and pathology found and recognized as such.

Careful patient setup and examination are a prerequisite of all arthroscopic procedures, as is careful portal placement. The arthroscope must also be used with care within the joint if iatrogenic chondral damage is to be avoided.

Although a systematic and sequential approach to the examination is described, as the surgeon becomes more experienced it is possible to deviate slightly from the protocol. Because a preoperative diagnosis must always be made there should be a region of suspected pathology. If this is quickly examined first the scrub nurse can be preparing the appropriate equipment while the rest of the examination is being completed. This can save crucial minutes when complex surgery is being contemplated.

The arthroscope is placed in the anterior lateral portal and will serve as the vantage point for the remainder of the illustrations. Looking from the anterior lateral portal through the patellofemoral joint, note the smoothness of the articular surfaces and the synovial lining.

We generally start the arthroscopic examination from the suprapatellas pouch and pull the arthroscope back towards the portal to see the patellofemoral joint. Great care must be taken to avoid gouging the articular surface while the arthroscope is in this position (Fig. 1.37).

The interval change from the previous figure is a slight move of the arthroscope medially. Further retraction of the arthroscope allows a more tangential view of the patellofemoral joint. By flexing the knee 20–30º the patella is engaged into the trochlear groove (Fig. 1.38).

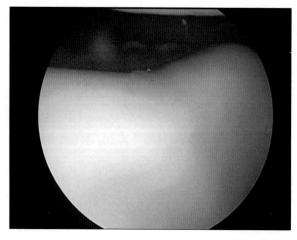

1.37

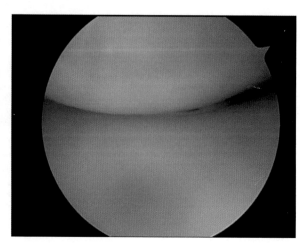

1.38

To move the arthroscope into the medial gutter one can proceed directly across the knee inferior to the patella. Again, great care must be exercised to protect the articular surface. A safer move is to go back into the suprapatellar pouch, pushing the edge of the arthroscope past the articular surface and moving down medially into the gutter. In the gutter, smooth synovium should blend into the posterior border of the medial femur. Look here when loose bodies are suspected (Fig. 1.39).

From here, move into the medial compartment by flexing the knee. Apply a valgus stress to the knee to open the medial compartment (Fig. 1.40).

An 18 g spinal needle is used to locate the proper position of the anterior medial portal. This should be above the medial meniscus and should enable the surgeon to reach the posterior aspect of the medial meniscus as well as the lateral compartment (Fig. 1.41).

Under direct vision a knife is used to enlarge the portal (Fig. 1.42).

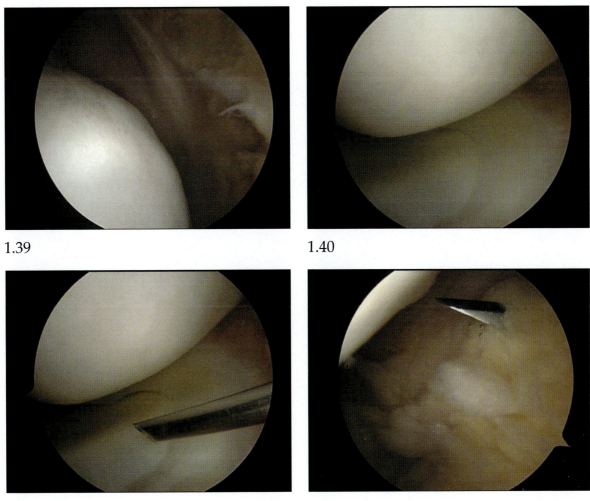

1.39

1.40

1.41

1.42

Insert a short blunt cannula to enlarge the portal. This will allow blood to flow out and can also be used as a working cannula for instruments (Fig. 1.43).

Once the medial portal is made, insert a probe to palpate the intra-articular structures. This palpation begins with the medial meniscus and articular cartilage of the medial femoral condyle and the medial tibial plateau (Fig. 1.44).

The undersurface of the meniscus must also be probed, as flaps and tears here may go unseen (Fig. 1.45).

The ligamentum mucosum is a structure of variable appearance. In this case it appears to be slightly fibrotic and connected to a bulbous fat pad. It can often make transfer from the medial to the lateral compartments difficult (Fig. 1.46).

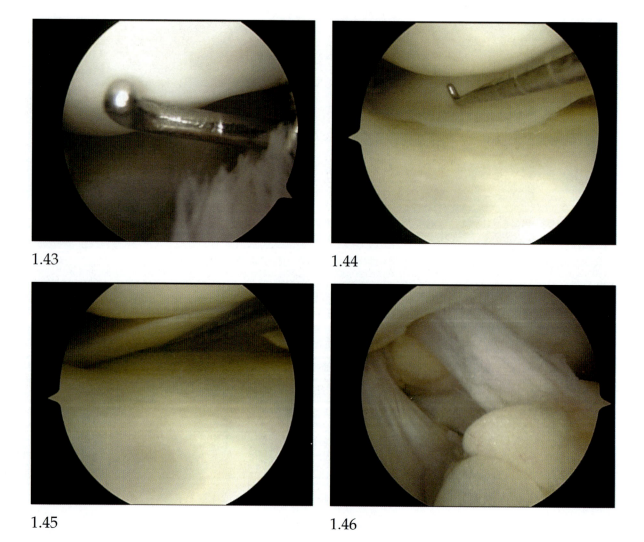

1.43

1.44

1.45

1.46

The ligamentum can easily be removed with a shaver and allows exposure of the ACL, as well as easier passage into the lateral compartment (Fig. 1.47).

Probe the ACL: in the uninjured ligament vessels can often be seen on its anterior surface. The ACL, PCL and the notch in general are best seen with the knee at 90º of flexion (Fig. 1.48).

With the knee now flexed and in a figure-of-four position, the lateral compartment is visualized. It is often easier to pass the probe into the posterior aspect of this compartment before the knee is put into the figure-of-four position (Fig. 1.49).

Use the probe to palpate the entire meniscus. The lateral meniscus separates from the capsule to allow the popliteal tendon to course up to the lateral epicondyle. This anatomic feature gives the lateral meniscus greater freedom and excursion when probing than is found with the medial meniscus (Fig. 1.50).

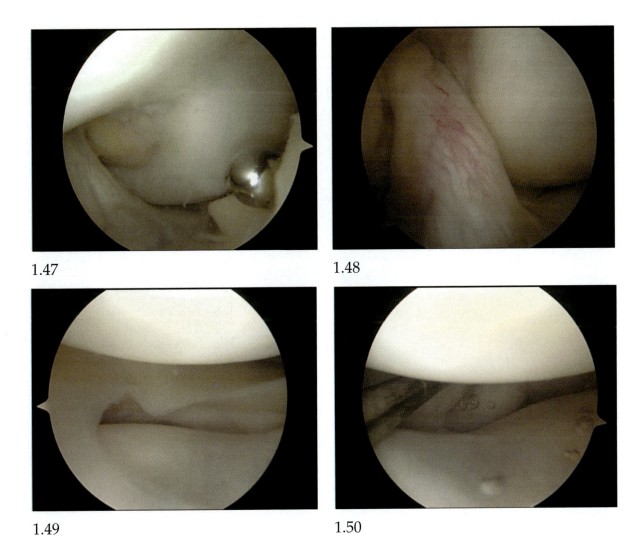

1.47

1.48

1.49

1.50

Carefully withdraw the arthroscope out of the lateral compartment and direct it across the lateral femoral condyle. This allows the anterior horn of the lateral meniscus to be visualized, although it may be necessary to rotate the light source to look down on the anterior horn (Fig. 1.51).

Simultaneously take the knee out of varus and place it in valgus. This will open up the lateral gutter. This is a favourite haven for loose bodies (Fig. 1.52).

Extend the knee as the arthroscope is advanced up the lateral gutter. Again, the smooth synovium blends with the lateral femur (Fig. 1.53).

The gutter gives way to the synovium covering the lateral patellar retinaculum. The retinaculum is difficult to evaluate when being distended by significant fluid pressure. This essentially brings the examination full circle. We do not routinely examine the posterior portions of the medial or lateral compartments. If there is any question, they should be carefully and thoroughly inspected as described in the section on creation of the posterior portals.

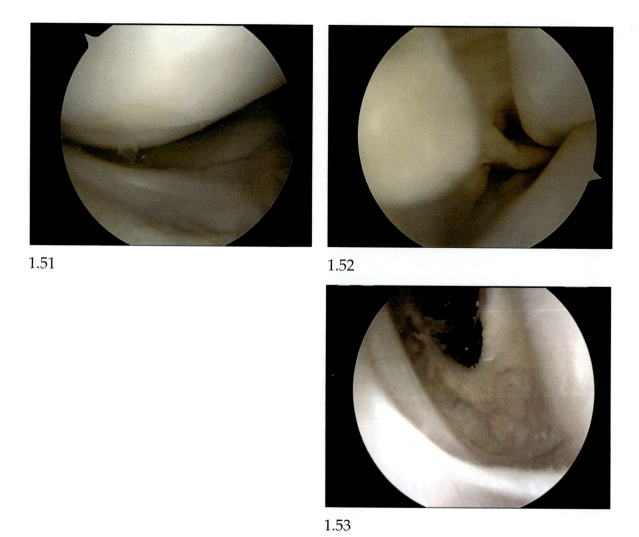

1.51

1.52

1.53

MENISCECTOMY

Partial meniscectomy is the staple procedure during knee arthroscopy. Meniscal excision can be very simple or very complex, and a range of instruments has been designed to make the procedure easier. All that is required for the vast majority of cases is a punch and a shaver, and it is possible to perform the debridement without the shaver if one is careful.

The important steps to be taken to reduce the need for a large number of instruments are first, patient positioning. Although this is a basic step, if the patient is not placed correctly on the table and the tourniquet is not in the correct place, the procedure will be more difficult.

Second, the placement of the anteromedial portal is crucial. The spinal needle must be used to plan the portal to allow the instruments to reach the tear at an appropriate angle. If the portal is placed correctly the punch will reach the tear and bite cleanly with the end. If the portal is incorrect either the instrument will not reach or it will be oblique to the tear and will not bite effectively. Using a trocar sleeve can make repeated passage of the instruments during the procedure much easier and reduce the risk of chondral damage. This is especially true for lateral meniscal tears.

Although many tears can be resected in this manner it may still not be possible to keep the punch perpendicular to all of a larger tear. These often propagate more anteriorly and may be more amenable to a side-cutting shaver. It is usually possible to obtain a good angle if the instrument and arthroscope are reversed, introducing the punch from the opposite portal (more commonly the anterolateral). The use of switching sticks makes swapping the instruments much easier.

Prepare and drape the patient. Make a standard anterolateral portal and inspect the whole joint to assess the work that needs to be done (Fig. 1.54).

Use an 18 g spinal needle to plan the anteromedial portal, as described previously. The tip of the needle must be able to reach all required areas (Fig. 1.55).

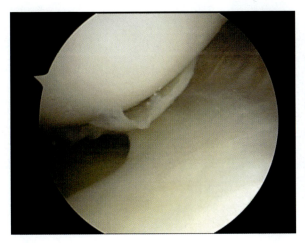

1.54

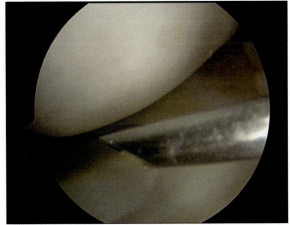

1.55

Make the anteromedial incision and insert a blunt trocar and sleeve (Fig. 1.56).

Remove the trocar and insert a hook probe (Fig. 1.57).

Use the probe to assess the meniscal tear (Fig. 1.58).

The torn meniscus can be removed using punches or a shaver. Often a combination of both instruments is required. If there is a clear, fine edge the shaver will work quickly. If the tissue is thicker or rolled over, the shaver should be replaced with the punch.

In this case the large flap is being minimized using the shaver (Fig. 1.59).

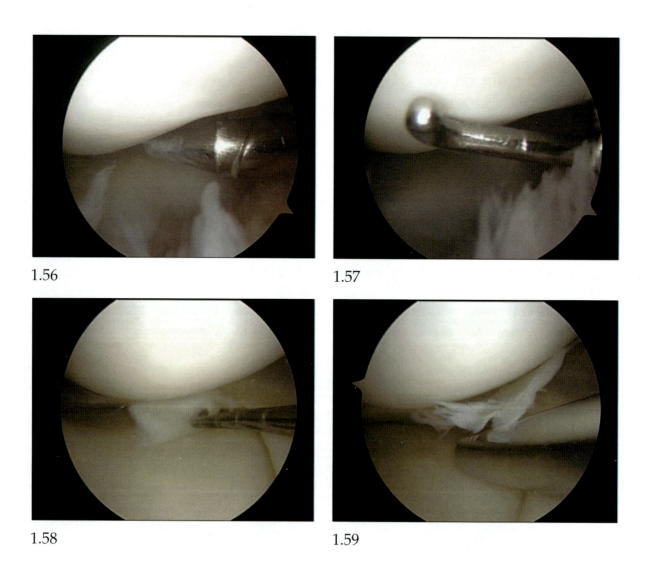

1.56

1.57

1.58

1.59

Introduce the punch. Work from one end of the tear to the other without removing the punch or the debris. After each bite move the punch along the meniscus without leaving a bridge of tissue. These are very difficult to smooth down later (Fig. 1.60).

Once sufficient tissue has been removed or the view has been obscured the shaver can be introduced to suction the debris and smooth the meniscus (Fig. 1.61).

Reinspect the meniscus, as tears are often more complex than they first appear. It may be necessary to reintroduce the punch or shaver to remove damaged meniscus that was not initially apparent (Fig. 1.62).

'Balance' the meniscus so that the free margin has no sharp edges (Fig. 1.63).

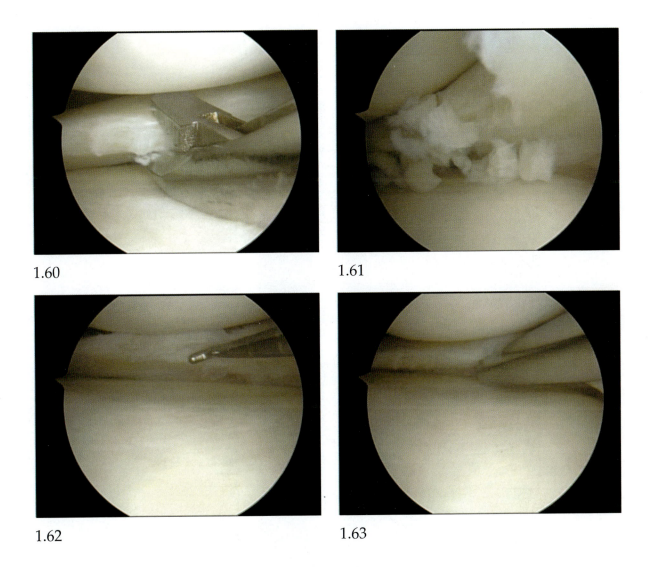

1.60

1.61

1.62

1.63

Reinspect the meniscus and the rest of the joint, and palpate any structures that have not previously been examined (Fig. 1.64).

Large flap tear

A large flap tear should be considered for treatment in the same manner as a bucket handle tear. The tear should first be probed to assess the full anatomy (Fig. 1.65).

Inspect the junction with the meniscus, as this is the region in which the resection will start (Fig. 1.66).

Using a small punch, start to transect the meniscus carefully at the neck, working from the leading to the trailing edge (Fig. 1.67).

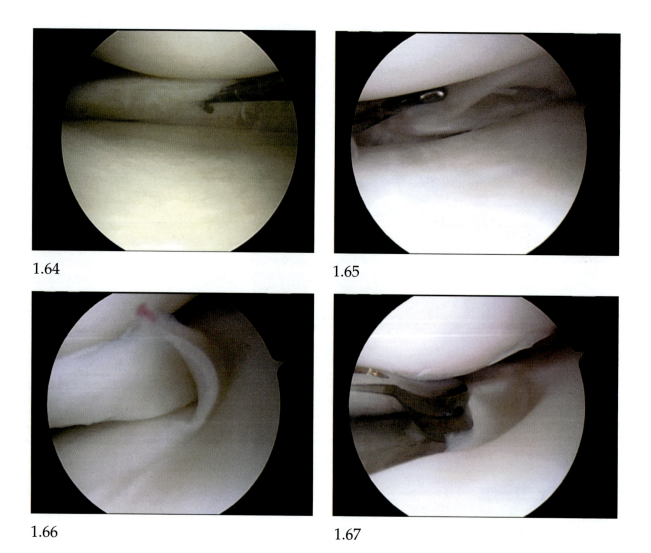

1.64

1.65

1.66

1.67

As the back of the meniscal flap is reached, leave a small rim of intact meniscus. This prevents a meniscal tear from becoming a loose body, which can be far more difficult to manage (Fig. 1.68).

Insert a grasper and, after a firm bite on the meniscal flap has been secured, withdraw the grasper, rotating it as it goes. The small meniscal rim will break and the flap will be extracted (Fig. 1.69).

A shaver can then be used to smooth the stump of the tear and balance the meniscus (Fig. 1.70).

The meniscus should then be probed to assess whether any further work should be done.

Bucket handle tear

A dislocated bucket handle tear will be evident early in the arthroscopic assessment as the torn meniscus lies in the intercondylar notch (Fig. 1.71).

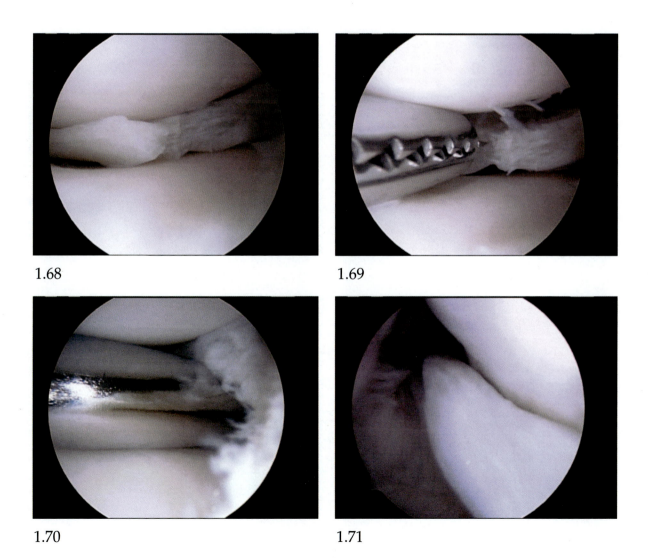

1.68

1.69

1.70

1.71

The meniscus should be assessed and consideration given to the possibility of meniscal repair. In this situation the tear is clearly chronic and the rim morphology is not suitable for repair (Fig. 1.72).

Identify the anterior edge of the bucket handle fragment. This should be detached as close to the anterior horn as possible using a small punch or arthroscopic scissors. Alternatively, the arthroscopic shaver can be used, but this often has difficulty if there is no free edge to work on (Fig. 1.73).

Introduce an arthroscopic shaver via the ipsilateral portal (in this case the anteromedial) and debride the flap, starting at the free end that has just been created. The suction will draw the flap into the shaver blade (Fig. 1.74).

Follow the flap to the posterior horn and smooth this. Sometimes this is easier with a small punch (Fig. 1.75).

Probe the meniscus and treat any further pathology as needed.

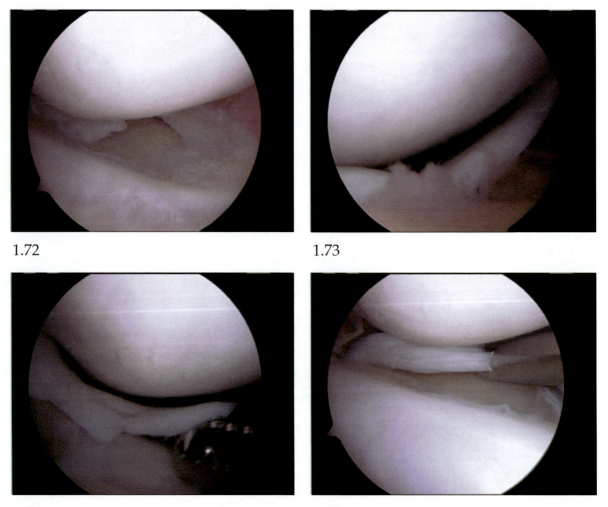

1.72

1.73

1.74

1.75

MENISCAL REPAIR

The majority of meniscal tears are not amenable to repair and should be resected. The indications for repair are increasing, and good healing rates are seen with red–red, red–white zone tears, tears in adolescents, and tears associated with ACL repairs. Repairs that are likely to fail are those in the white–white zone, isolated medial meniscal tears, and those in ACL-deficient unstable knees. Lateral tears seem to have a better healing rate than the medial side, and the attempt at repair seems justified given the appalling results of lateral meniscectomy.

Meniscal repair should therefore be considered in all patients in whom the torn meniscus can be reduced satisfactorily. Consideration must be given to compliance with a postoperative regimen that will include bracing, restricted motion and limited weightbearing.

As with all aspects of arthroscopic surgery there are a multitude of implants available to effect meniscal repair. Some are good, some have poor results. The most basic technique is that of suturing the meniscus. There are essentially two ways of achieving this, the outside-in technique and the inside-out technique. We favour, and have described here, the inside-out because it is comparatively simple, safe, and requires only a basic set of instruments. It does, however, prevent the surgeon from repairing posterior tears, for which arrows are more suitable. The authors would advise that the surgeon has available a range of devices (sutures and arrows) to maximize the chances of successful repair.

Prepare and drape the patient as for routine knee arthroscopy. If a meniscal lesion is suspected, ensure that there is adequate access to both the posteromedial and posterolateral aspects of the knee. This may mean moving the contralateral leg further across the operating table.

Introduce the arthroscope via an anterolateral portal and inspect the whole knee as routine. Treat any other pathology in sequence. If the anterior cruciate ligament (ACL) is to be repaired it is advisable to repair the meniscus first.

Once a meniscal tear has been identified the decision whether to debride or repair must be made. There are a number of criteria that should be met, and these are outside the scope of this book.

Assess the extent of the tear using the hook probe. If the tear is of the bucket handle variety ensure that it can be reduced before attempting to repair it, as chronic tears may become fixed in the 'dislocated' position (Fig. 1.76).

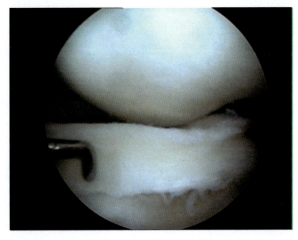

1.76

Use a shaver or a rasp to debride the meniscosynovial junction throughout the extent of the tear. Rasps are available which will debride both the meniscus and the synovium, but these can sometimes be difficult to introduce into the knee. The shaver is easier to introduce but may have difficulty reaching all areas and both sides (Fig. 1.77).

The simplest and cheapest technique for meniscal repair is the inside-out. In this the sutures are passed out through the meniscus to exit through the skin. The skin is incised and the suture ends tied down over the capsule. The technique is clearly limited to the body and anterior horn of the meniscus, as a needle exiting posteriorly places the neurovascular structures at risk.

The inside-out technique uses zone-specific cannulas. The point of reference for the cannulas is from the surgeon's perspective, regardless of whether a left or right knee is involved. For example, a right posterior cannula is used for a right posterior horn medial meniscal repair. A left posterior cannula is used for a right knee, lateral meniscal repair (Fig. 1.78).

Specially designed sutures for meniscal repair (with the needles attached) expedite the procedure. We routinely use 2/0 PDS sutures (Fig. 1.79).

Introduce the cannula via the contralateral portal. For a medial meniscal tear this will mean switching the instruments so that the arthroscope is in the anteromedial portal.

It is easier to perform the repair working from posterior to anterior; however, for the purposes of illustration suture insertion into the anterior meniscus will be shown.

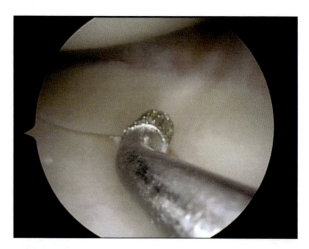

1.77

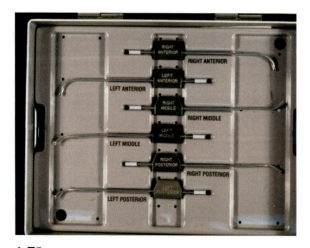

1.78

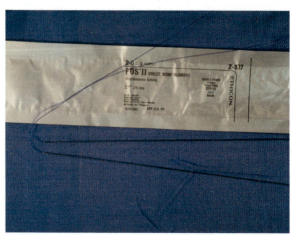

1.79

Introduce the cannula and place it in position over the meniscus. The needle is then inserted by the assistant and advanced until 1–2 mm protrude from the tip of the cannula (Fig. 1.80).

The cannula and needle are then advanced until the needle enters the meniscus in the desired position (Fig. 1.81).

The assistant then advances the needle through the meniscus. The progress must be monitored and the exit point observed carefully. Once the tip of the needle penetrates the skin it can be pulled using a haemostat (Fig. 1.82).

Once the full length of the needle has been pulled through the meniscus insert the second needle and advance it as before. Reposition the needle tip to create the limb of the suture. This may be in a horizontal or a vertical orientation (Fig. 1.83).

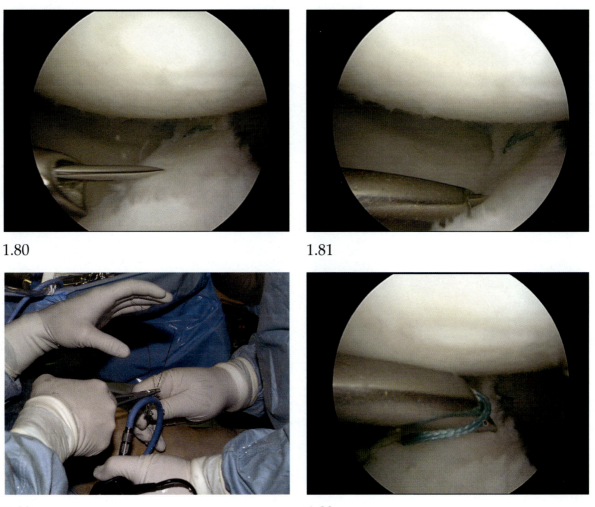

1.80

1.81

1.82

1.83

Advance the second needle through the skin as before (Fig. 1.84).

Repeat the process round the meniscus until all sutures are in place (Fig. 1.85).

Once all of the sutures have been inserted the external view should be as in this external view of the medial side of the knee, showing the meniscal sutures exiting through the skin (Fig. 1.86).

Separate the limbs of the sutures into an anterior and a posterior bundle. Make an incision which is centred between the sutures (Fig. 1.87).

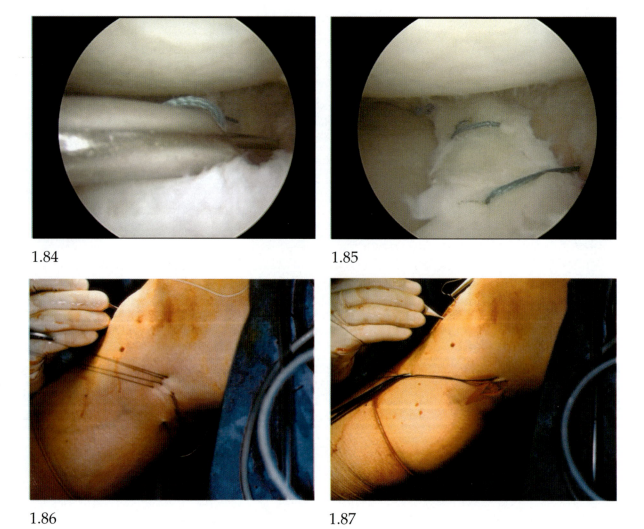

1.84

1.85

1.86

1.87

Blunt dissect down to the capsule. This will enable the sutures to be pulled into the incision and tied over the capsule. Care must be taken not to involve the saphenous nerve in any of the sutures (Fig. 1.88).

For a lateral meniscal repair the exit point of the sutures is close to the common peroneal nerve as it winds round the fibula neck. It is therefore not safe to pass the sutures blindly through the skin.

Mark out the position of the anatomical landmarks on the skin (Fig. 1.89).

Make an incision between the iliotibial band and the biceps tendon (Fig. 1.90).

Using a finger, blunt dissect down to the lateral head of gastrocnemius and reflect this away from the posterolateral capsule (Fig. 1.91).

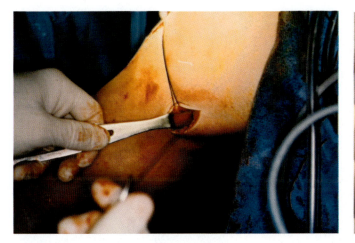

1.88

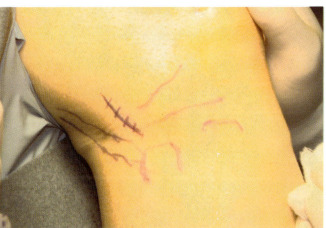

1.89

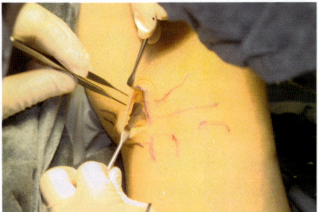

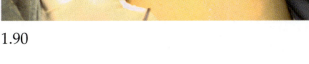

1.90

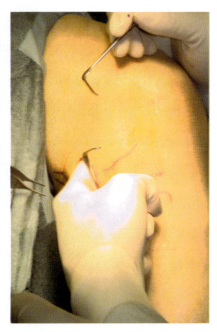

1.91

Place a meniscus retractor or paediatric vaginal speculum or a spoon deep in the wound anterior to the lateral head of gastrocnemius. This will help to catch the needle and protect the peroneal nerve (Fig. 1.92).

Pass the sutures in the same fashion as for the medial side. Pay careful attention to the exit site of the needle. It may be necessary to redirect the sutures if they are not being caught in the retractor/spoon. As each pair of suture limbs is passed, secure them with a haemostat (Fig. 1.93).

Once all the lateral sutures have been passed tie them down over the capsule in the manner described for the medial side (Fig. 1.94).

In both the medial and the lateral repair reinspect the meniscus after the sutures have been tied, and then close the skin by whatever means is preferred.

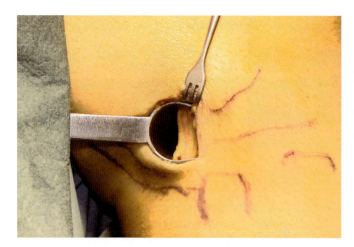

1.92

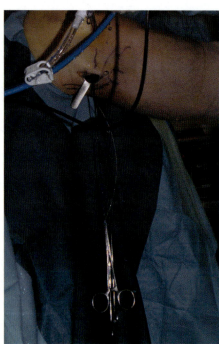

1.93

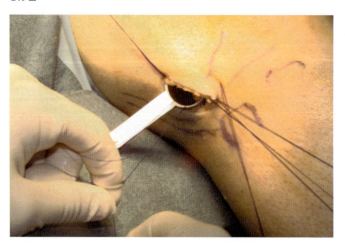

1.94

LATERAL RELEASE

Patellar maltracking is a common cause of anterior knee pain. In many cases part of the aetiology is tight lateral retinacular structures. The diagnosis can be suggested by a number of preoperative steps, including examination and investigations such as X-ray and CT scans. During the arthroscopic examination the patellar position should be assessed. The position is not a true representation of the normal anatomy, as the knee joint is distended with irrigation fluid. However, if the surgeon has an appreciation of normal patellar position (through experience of routine examination) it is possible to determine that a patella is placed laterally with respect to the trochlear groove.

Lateral retinacular release is an accepted method of allowing the patella to return to the trochlear groove and hopefully to track normally. There is debate as to the long-term effectiveness, but for many patients significant relief of pain is obtained.

It is important to obtain a good view and appreciate the relevant anatomy before the release is undertaken. This can be difficult to learn, as by necessity the instruments have to be reversed and the arthroscope introduced through the anteromedial portal. Rehearsing the movement with a probe or switching stick is invaluable when one is learning the procedure.

As the release approaches the lateral portal it is advisable to reintroduce the shaver to obtain a clear view. Occasionally it is necessary to continue the release beyond the antero-lateral portal (depending on the portal position). In this case care should be taken that the lateral meniscus and the patellar tendon are not damaged.

Occasionally it may be necessary to undertake a revision lateral release. In these cases it is not advisable to use the diathermy blade as the tissues are not normal and it is possible to cause a full-thickness burn without realizing. Use a banana blade and introduce the diathermy afterwards to coagulate any visible bleeding vessels.

Prepare and drape the patient as for routine knee arthroscopy. Perform a diagnostic arthroscopy and treat any other pathology within the knee.

Assess the patella for position and tracking. This is often easier with the arthroscope in the anteromedial portal. Because of the fluid distension of the knee the position of the patella is not absolute but relative, and only experience will guide the surgeon as to the extent of patellar maltracking (Fig. 1.95).

If it has not already been done, switch the arthroscope to the anteromedial portal. This may be easier using a switching stick, which also reduces the risk of chondral damage during the exchange (Fig. 1.96).

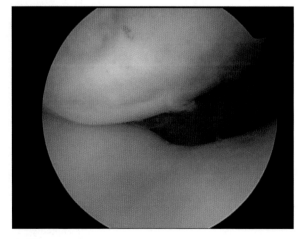

1.95

Introduce a switching stick through the anterolateral portal to 'rehearse' the release. It may be necessary to alter the arthroscope's position, so ensure that the tip of the switching stick can be seen throughout the 'procedure' (Fig. 1.97).

The release can be performed with a blade or diathermy. The advantage of diathermy is that bleeding can be controlled. The risk is of skin necrosis. This is of particular concern in revision cases, and diathermy is not recommended for these (Fig. 1.98).

Start the release level with the superior pole of the patella and continue it to the antero-lateral portal. The release needs to be low enough that the patellar tendon is not being cut (Fig. 1.99).

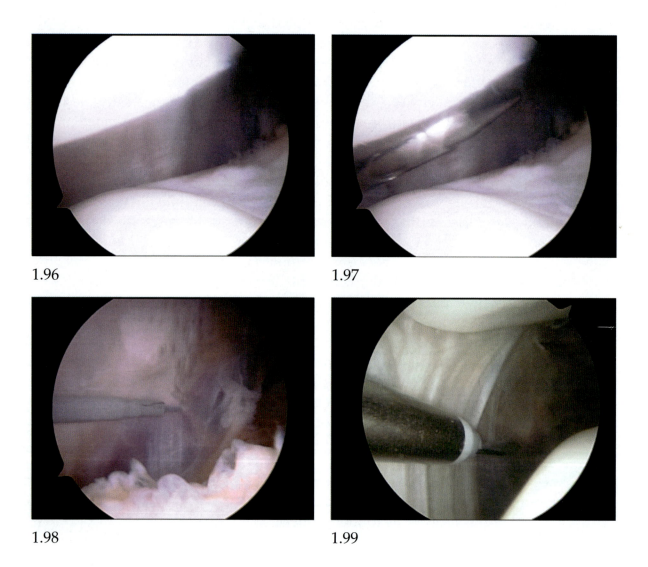

1.96

1.97

1.98

1.99

Develop the release through the layers of tissue until fat is seen. Sometimes it is necessary to perform an incomplete release along the length and then return to the proximal end (Fig. 1.100).

Once the tissues have been divided from the proximal pole to the portal site, reinspect the free edges for bleeding points (Fig. 1.101).

Assess patellar mobility to determine whether the release is sufficient or if a further procedure should be performed (Fig. 1.102).

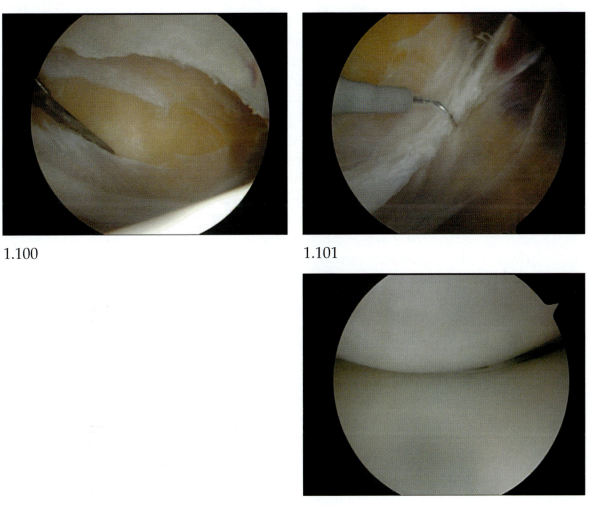

1.100

1.101

1.102

VASTUS MEDIALIS OBLIQUUS PLICATION

Patellar maltracking is a common cause of anterior knee pain and is notoriously difficult to diagnose and treat. The diagnosis is made using a combination of the history, examination and special investigations, which will not be discussed here. During arthroscopy the position of the patella in relation to the trochlear groove can be assessed. Because the knee is distended with irrigation fluid the tracking is not truly normal. However, with experience it is possible to appreciate the difference between normal and abnormal (lateral) tracking. The treatment of patellar maltracking is controversial and the authors do not claim to have all of the answers. What we have seen, however, is that lateral retinacular release will often allow the patella to sit better in the trochlear groove and will improve the tracking.

In a small number of cases the patella will continue to lie off the lateral femoral condyle despite an adequate retinacular release. These patients may benefit from plication of the vastus medialis obliquus (VMO). Again this technique is not universally accepted, but does appear to improve tracking and does result in a reduction of pain for many patients. It is argued that the tissues stretch out over time, and this may well be true in some cases; however, at the time of surgery it is not possible to predict which ones will fail. If the procedure is performed correctly there is little morbidity and later surgical procedures are not excluded should they become necessary.

It is important first to perform an adequate lateral release and to reassess the patellar tracking. The patella must also be reassessed during and after the VMO plication. It is essential that the VMO is not overtightened, as this can result in increased contact pressures between either the patella and the trochlear groove or between the medial facet of the patella and the medial femoral condyle.

There are a number of different techniques described for VMO plication. The one we describe here is simple to undertake and has produced consistent and reliable results in our practice.

Prepare and drape the knee in the standard fashion. Introduce the arthroscope via an anterolateral portal and inspect the knee. Assess patellar tracking as described in the section on lateral release. It may be beneficial to switch the arthroscope to the anteromedial portal for this.

The first step in improving patellar tracking is the release of the tight lateral retinacular structures – the lateral release, discussed in the previous chapter. Patellar tracking should be reassessed after this (Fig. 1.103).

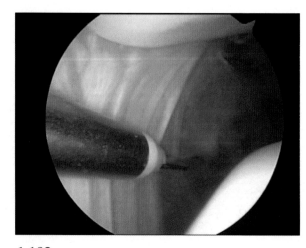

1.103

If the patella still tracks laterally a medial plication may be beneficial. Also, inspect the medial facet of the patella carefully. If there is chondral damage affecting the medial facet a medial plication may make the patient symptomatically worse (Fig. 1.104).

Use a number 2 non-absorbable suture on a wide-radius cutting needle. Insert the first suture just medial to the medial edge of the patella near the superior pole. Try to ensure that the needle enters the joint perpendicular to the soft tissues, and use the curve of the needle to direct it (Fig. 1.105).

Watch the needle arthroscopically and guide it so that the suture runs perpendicular to the long axis of the leg (Fig. 1.106).

Aim to take a 2–2.5 cm bite of tissue. This should be dictated largely by the radius of curvature of the needle. Once the needle has exited the skin, secure the ends with a haemostat (Fig. 1.107).

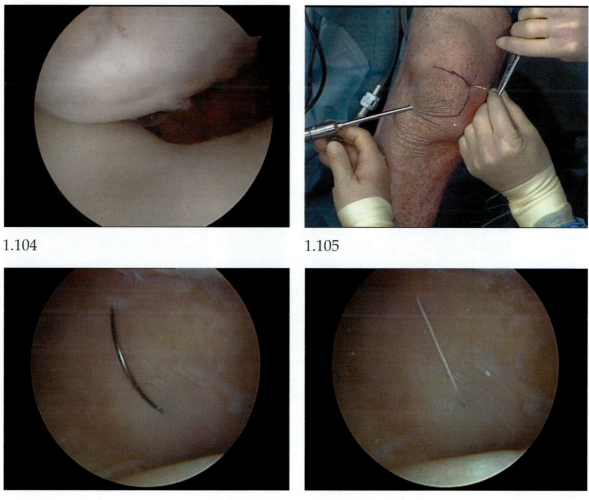

1.104

1.105

1.106

1.107

Place a second suture 1–1.5 cm distal to the first (Fig. 1.108).

Again, watch the progress of the suture arthroscopically so that the exit point is parallel to the first and secure it with a second haemostat (Fig. 1.109).

Place a further two sutures, making a total of four. All of these should be parallel when viewed from within the joint (Fig. 1.110).

Make a skin incision in Langer's lines between the anterior and posterior limbs of the sutures (Fig. 1.111).

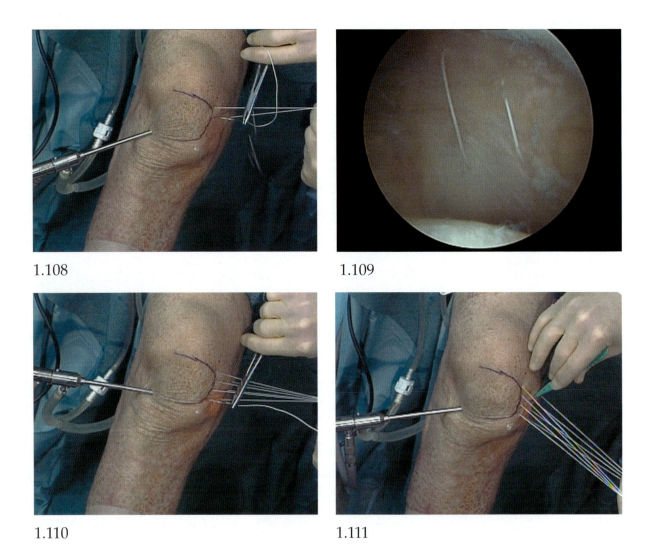

1.108

1.109

1.110

1.111

Blunt dissect using a finger or haemostat until the capsule is reached. The saphenous vein and nerve should be posterior to the sutures, but blunt dissection will ensure that the sutures are not tied over them (Fig. 1.112).

Tie each of the sutures in turn. We usually start with the proximal suture and work distally. The tension can be estimated by watching the position of the patella arthroscopically. Remember that the tension and hence the contact pressure will increase as the knee is flexed. It is therefore important not to make the sutures too tight. If it is not possible to realign the patella using this technique do not force it but consider a distal patellar realignment procedure (Fig. 1.113).

Re-examine patellar tracking before closing the wound in layers (Fig. 1.114).

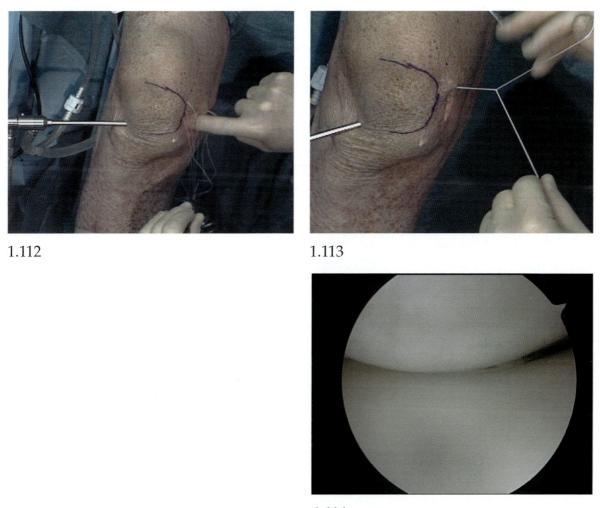

1.112

1.113

1.114

PLICA EXCISION

The medial parapatellar plica is present in 25% of the normal population and is commonly bilateral. Occasionally it can become inflamed and thickened, causing anteromedial knee pain. In some patients surgical excision may be necessary.

The plica is often seen as the arthroscope is moved from the suprapatellar pouch into the medial compartment, and may obstruct the passage of the arthroscope if it is large. Often it is easier to obtain a clear view of a plica as the arthroscope is reintroduced into the superior compartment of the knee after the lateral joint has been inspected.

Debridement of a plica often necessitates the removal of some of the anterior fat pad, which results in bleeding. For this reason routine use of a tourniquet is recommended. It is sometimes difficult for the shaver to obtain a purchase on the edge of the plica, and it may be necessary to use a punch to create a free edge for the shaver to work on. Frequently the anteromedial portal is in such a position that it is not possible to obtain a satisfactory angle to work on the plica. If this is the case, introduce a blunt trocar and sheath through the portal site and redirect the trocar through the capsule, creating a new portal position which allows you to work on the plica. The sheath is then left in situ to guide the passage of the instruments.

Prepare and drape the knee in the standard fashion. Introduce the arthroscope via the anterolateral portal and inspect the knee as usual. If a symptomatic plica is suspected the capsule overlying the medial femoral condyle should be inspected.

A plica will be seen as a crescent-shaped band of tissue overlying the medial femoral condyle. In many cases it will be seen as a thin tissue paper-like structure, but if it has been traumatized it may become a thick hard band (Fig. 1.115).

Often the plica is difficult to see initially as the arthroscope is passed into the medial compartment. If there is a ligamentum mucosum this will tend to tether the patellar tendon and make a good view more difficult. If the ligamentum is released as part of the inspection of the knee the plica may become more obvious when the arthroscope is reintroduced into the suprapatellar pouch.

As the knee is flexed the plica can be seen to come into contact with the medial femoral condyle (Fig. 1.116).

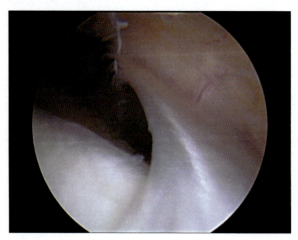

1.115

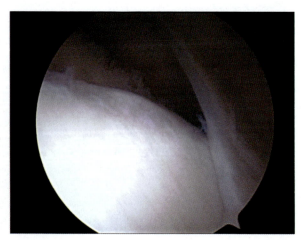

1.116

Introduce a shaver through the anteromedial portal. If the fat pad is large, or there is proliferative tissue behind the patellar tendon, it may be necessary to debride this before the plica can be clearly seen (Fig. 1.117).

If the plica is relatively thin it can be removed easily with the shaver (Fig. 1.118).

Continue the debridement back to the capsule. Be careful not to be too aggressive inferiorly, as the medial meniscus can be close (Fig. 1.119).

If the plica is very thick it may be necessary to use a punch to create an edge for the shaver to work on (Fig. 1.120).

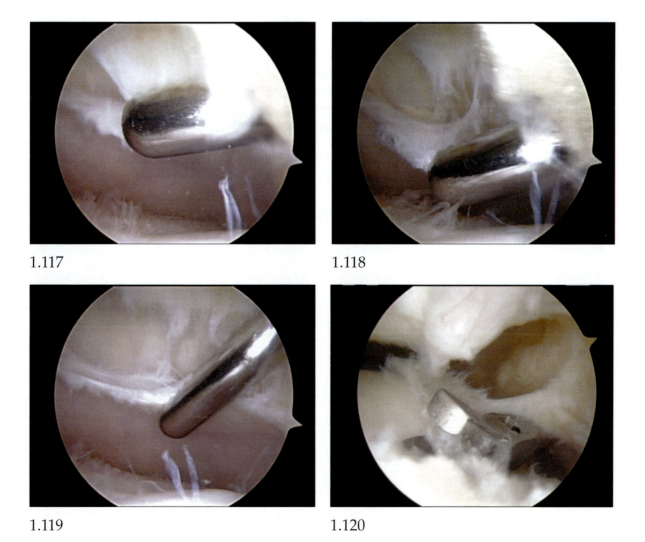

1.117

1.118

1.119

1.120

At the end of the procedure there should be no tissue impinging on the medial femoral condyle. If extensive fat pad debridement has been performed it is advisable to introduce the diathermy and cauterize any obvious bleeding vessels (Fig. 1.121).

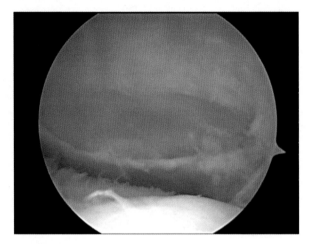

1.121

CHONDROPLASTY

Chondral damage is frequently seen during knee arthroscopy. Fortunately total-thickness cartilage loss is seen less frequently. However, what may appear on first inspection to be partial thickness may become total thickness once an adequate debridement has been done.

The treatment of discrete, full-thickness articular cartilage loss is controversial and there is no 'right' answer. Microfracture aims to reduce pain by replacing the articular cartilage with fibrocartilage. Second-look arthroscopy has demonstrated visually satisfying results, although there is no good correlation with pain reduction. More complex procedures, such as osteochondral autografting and chondrocyte transplantation, have reported similar results.

Microfracture is relatively simple to perform, cheap, has little associated morbidity, and does not preclude later, more complex intervention should it become necessary. It is important, however, to ensure that the treated area is not loaded while the fibrocartilage matures, as there is a risk of displacement.

In most cases it is possible to undertake microfracture using the standard anteromedial and anterolateral portals. If these do not allow perpendicular access it is essential to make additional portals as required. If the holes are not perpendicular to the articular surface there is a risk that the bone will fracture, leaving a larger bony defect and a loose body within the joint. Similarly, it is important not to make the holes too close together.

Prepare and drape the patient. Make a standard anterolateral portal and inspect the whole joint to assess the work that needs to be done.

Identify the lesion and assess the extent of the potential defect. Often, as the loose edge is resected the defect becomes larger than was first anticipated. In this case the lesion is in the lateral aspect of the medial femoral condyle (Fig. 1.122).

Resect the free edges until they are stable. This may be done with a combination of punches and shaver. The suction punch is useful here as it has a very small inferior lip that reduces the remaining free edge, and the suction removes debris. It may be necessary to switch portals to improve access, as in this case (Fig. 1.123).

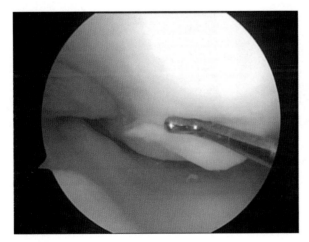

1.122

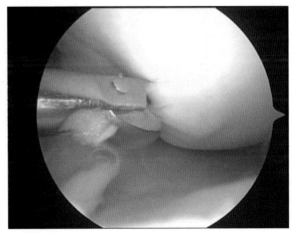

1.123

Attempt to make the edges as perpendicular to the subchondral surface as possible. This can be difficult in smaller lesions such as the one here (Fig. 1.124).

Insert the chondroplasty pick. The pick should be perpendicular to the base of the lesion. It may be possible to achieve this using the working portal or a particular angle of pick. If this is not possible from a standard portal, it may be necessary to create an accessory portal (Fig. 1.125).

Have the assistant tap the pick with a mallet, driving it 2–3 mm into the subchondral bone (Fig. 1.126).

Create additional holes approximately 2–3 mm apart (Fig. 1.127).

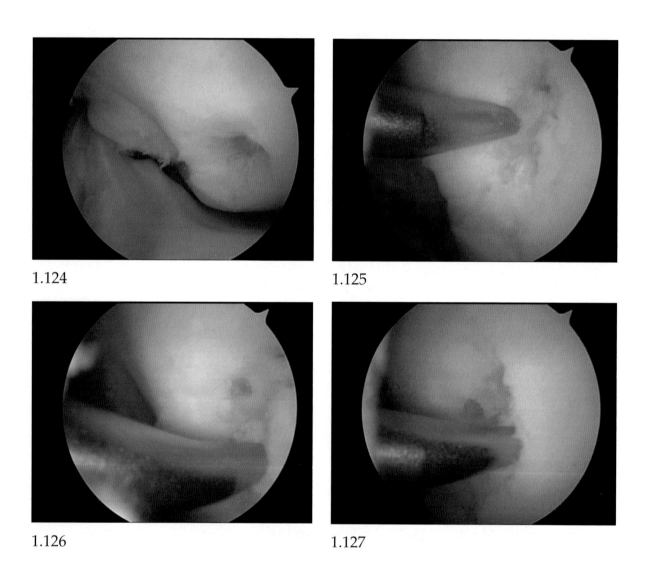

1.124

1.125

1.126

1.127

If the area of chondral loss is extensive the same principles apply. The loose cartilage is removed and the edges are left perpendicular to the subchondral bone. The pick is introduced perpendicular to the surface (Fig. 1.128).

With a large lesion it is best to work to a pattern, as opposed to randomly inserting the pick into the lesion. This ensures that the maximum area is covered without the creation of narrow bone bridges. In this case the pick has been moved circumferentially before completing the central portion of the defect (Fig. 1.129).

At the completion of the case adequate bone bridges must be left to prevent subchondral collapse (Fig 1.130).

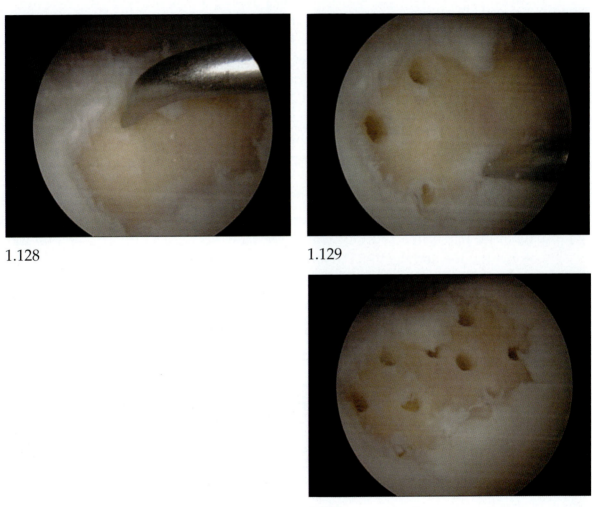

1.128

1.129

1.130

44

ANTERIOR CRUCIATE LIGAMENT RECONSTRUCTION

Reconstruction of the anterior cruciate ligament (ACL) is now a routine part of arthroscopic surgery and the results are improving significantly. There are three different constructs commonly used to replace the ruptured ligament: bone–patellar tendon–bone, hamstring and allograft. There are advantages and disadvantages to each, and ultimately there is little to choose from between them. What is more important is the correct placement of the graft in relation to the original ACL insertions, adequate tension of the graft, and suitable fixation on both the femoral and the tibial sides.

In this chapter the preparation of all three graft types is described, together with the methods of tunnel preparation and graft passage. There are so many techniques of graft fixation that it is beyond the scope of this book to describe them all. We have described our preferred methods of graft fixation; however, as we have stated before, there are alternatives and new devices are coming on to the market daily. As long as the fixation method is reproducible, secure, and will remain so during graft incorporation, the precise method is not as important as the surgical skill.

A number of neurovascular structures are at risk during the various incisions used during the procedure, and attention should be paid to these.

Hamstring graft preparation

With the patient in a supine position on the operating table, the foot is dropped and the patient prepared in a routine fashion for arthroscopy. The inferior pole of the patella, the patellar tendon and the tibial tubercle may be marked. Palpate the pes anserinus to identify the proper location of the harvesting incision (Fig. 1.131).

The harvest incision coincides with the appropriate location for the tibial tunnel. This incision is approximately 1–1.5 cm medial and approximately 2 cm distal to the tibial tubercle (Fig. 1.132).

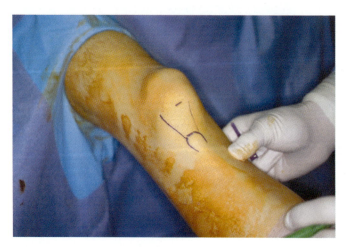

1.131

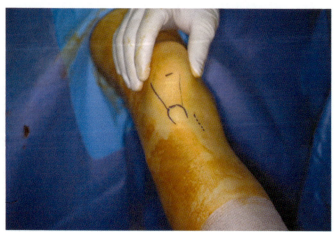

1.132

Incise the skin and subcutaneous tissue with a knife. Extend the incision down through the periosteum. Superficial to the periosteum is the insertion of the pes anserinus. Separate the pes insertion from the periosteum (Fig. 1.133).

Elevate the pes anserinus to inspect the undersurface of the sartorius fascia. It is important at this stage to find the semitendinosus and gracilis tendons on the underside or bone side of this fascia (Fig. 1.134).

The tendons can be very difficult to identify from outside the fascia, but very easy to identify from inside this fascial layer. Lift this layer and view it from the bone side, instead of from outside (Fig. 1.135).

Viewing from inside, a raphe can be identified between the semitendinosus, which is most inferior, and the gracilis, which is more superior. Dissection scissors can then be used to separate these tendons from the undersurface of the sartorius (Fig. 1.136).

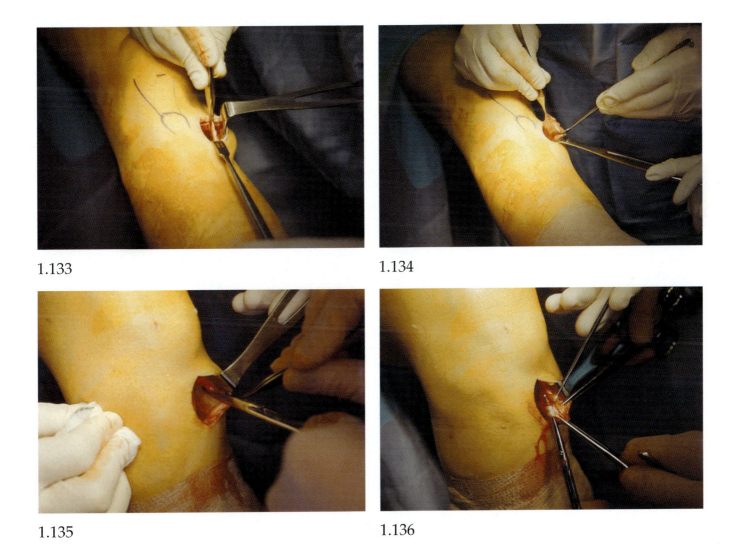

1.133

1.134

1.135

1.136

Once the ends of the tendons have been identified, place no. 5 Ethibond sutures in a modified Krackow-type pattern or whip-stitch through the tendon at its tendinous end (Fig. 1.137).

Both tendons are shown in the wound, with the raphe having been incised to allow their partial separation (Fig. 1.138).

Using a pair of dissection scissors, separate the semitendinosus and gracilis at the pes anserinus to the point where they are anatomically separate tendons (Fig. 1.139).

It should be noted that there are occasionally adherent bands running from the semi-tendinosus especially, but occasionally from the gracilis to the medial head of the gastrocnemius. These need to be divided prior to passing the tendon stripper. If they are not released before harvesting then there is a significant risk of amputating the hamstring at the level of the gastrocnemius connection (Fig. 1.140).

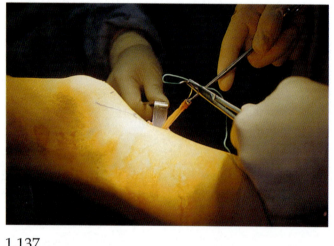

1.137

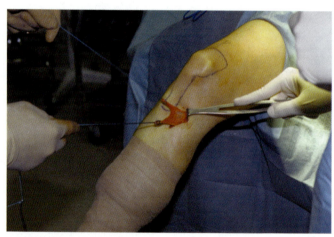

1.138

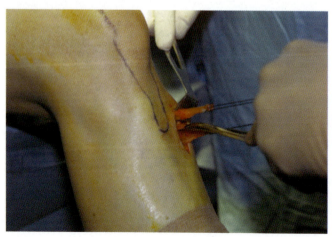

1.139

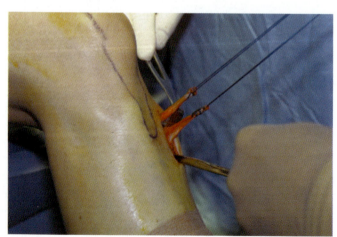

1.140

One method of performing this task is to feed the suture and tendon end through a short arthroscopic trocar sleeve once the suture has been placed in the tendon (Fig. 1.141).

Flex the knee to 90º and advance the trocar proximally as far as it will go. This will break down any adhesions and confirms that sufficient length will be obtained when the tendon stripper is used (Fig. 1.142).

Flexing the knee at 90° allows easy and atraumatic harvesting of the tendon. With the knee flexed, pass the tendon stripper up the tendon. It is important to maintain good tension on the tendon to avoid early tendon amputation (Fig. 1.143).

When the tendon/muscle is cut proximally, the tension is automatically reduced and the tendon is removed (Fig. 1.144).

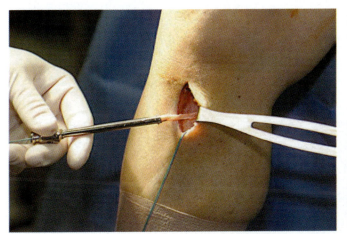

1.141

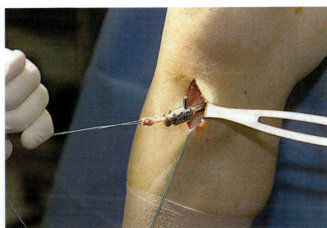

1.142

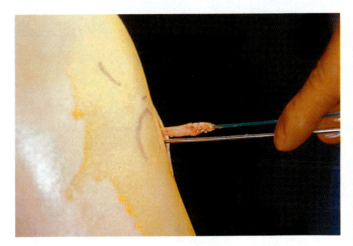

1.143

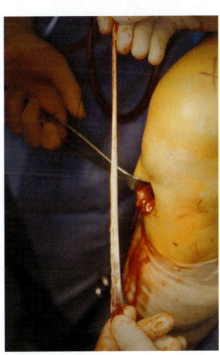

1.144

Once the tendons are harvested, take them to the back table and remove the muscle from the proximal portion. Place a no. 5 Ethibond whip-type stitch in the end of the tendon to provide a mechanism to tension the graft (Fig. 1.145).

An Endobutton with integral loop is routinely used for femoral fixation in our practice. The construct comes in standard loop lengths and reduces the risk of knot slippage in the older Endobutton constructs. This is applied when the femoral tunnel has been drilled and measured (Fig. 1.146).

Once the tendons have been looped through the Endobutton the construct can be attached to an ACL preparation board. In this device the Endobutton is secured at one end and the free sutures at the other. This enables the tendon lengths to be equalized and the construct to be 'pretensioned' (Fig. 1.147).

Finally, the tendon is marked at a point which is equal to the length of the femoral tunnel plus the length of the Endobutton and loop. This means that when the mark passes into the femoral tunnel the Endobutton should flip easily (Fig. 1.148).

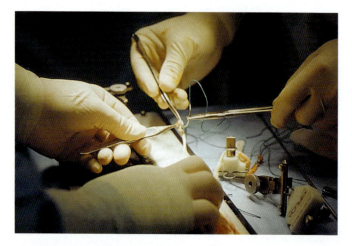

1.145

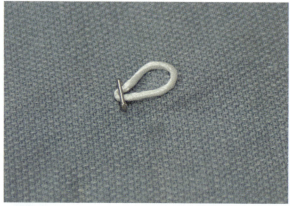

1.146

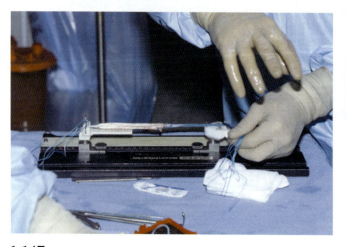

1.147

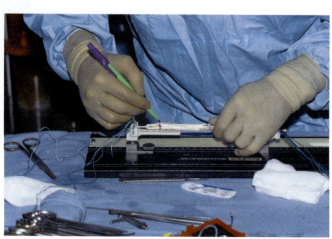

1.148

Allograft preparation

Graft preparation for allografts begin with reconstitution of the graft. At Tuckahoe Orthopaedics and Orthopaedic Research of Virginia only freeze-dried allografts are used to ensure the patient's safety. The graft is stored in a clear bottle and is reconstituted with antibiotic saline (Fig. 1.149).

Remove the fascia lata allograft from the jar and unroll it into a sheet (Fig. 1.150).

All ACL grafts, bone–tendon–bone, hamstring or allograft, are prepared on an ACL graft board. We routinely use one produced by Acufex.

The graft is attached to the board via two alligator clamps. It may be necessary to supplement this with haemostats (Fig. 1.151).

Roll the graft tightly into a tube, leaving the corners attached to the alligator clips (Fig. 1.152).

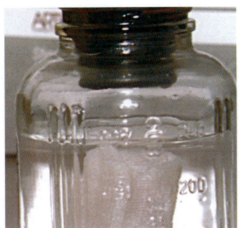

1.149

1.150

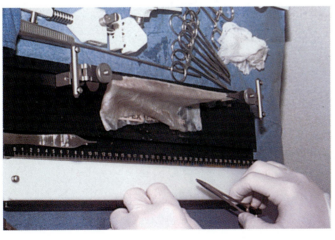

1.151

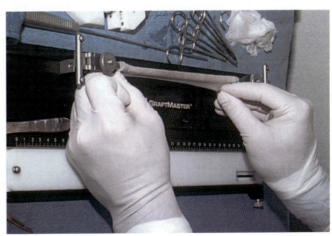

1.152

Suture the edge of the graft using a 2/0 Vicryl suture to prevent the rolled tube from unrolling. This suture is tied securely at each end (Fig. 1.153).

Place a no. 5 Ethibond suture through each end of the graft in a modified Krackow or whip-stitch fashion to capture the graft end securely. These will be used to pass the graft through the knee and may be required as a means of alternative fixation, and so they must be secure (Fig. 1.154).

Pull firmly on both sutures to confirm that they are firmly placed into the ends of the graft, and that the graft itself is competent (Fig. 1.155).

Loop (double) the allograft and size it. It takes several cases to realize how large the graft will be as it is rolled. Normally a 5 × 18 cm sheet of fascia lata allograft will produce a 10–12 mm graft after rolling and looping (doubling) (Fig. 1.156.

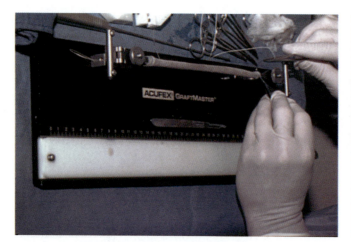

1.153

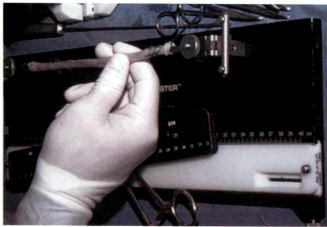

1.154

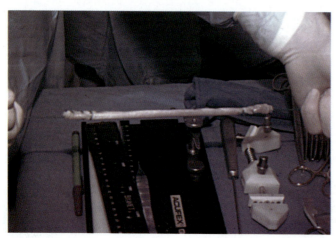

1.155

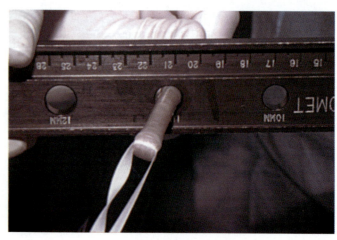

1.156

Sizing sleeves may also be used to size the graft so that the appropriate-diameter drill bit can be chosen to create the bone tunnels (Fig. 1.157).

Once the graft preparation is completed, cover it with a saline-soaked gauze to keep it moist while the intra-articular portion of the procedure is completed.

In our practice the Endobutton is used routinely and will be attached after the femoral tunnel has been drilled and measured. The technique of preparing the graft for insertion is described in the section on hamstring autograft preparation (Fig. 1.146).

Bone–tendon–bone preparation

The patient setup and preparation are identical to those for the other techniques of ACL reconstruction. Because of the greater amount of soft tissue dissection the use of a tourniquet is recommended.

The prepatellar skin and bursae can be injected with marcaine plus epinephrine (adrenaline) to limit bleeding (Fig. 1.158).

Draw the anatomy of the patellar tendon graft with a skin marker. Make a linear incision directly over the patellar tendon (Fig. 1.159).

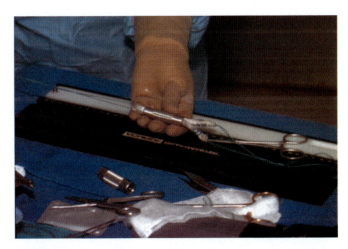

1.157

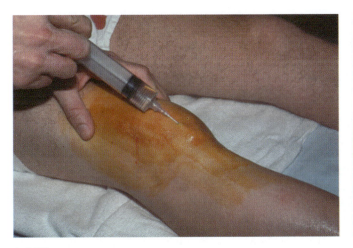

1.158

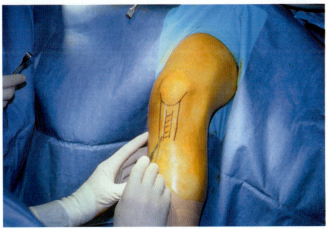

1.159

Incise the skin from the inferior pole of the patella to the tibial tubercle. The incision must extend far enough distally to expose the entry site of the tibial tunnel. Carry the incision down to the depth of the patellar tendon. Expose the entire patellar tendon and mobilize it so that the central third can be harvested. Two centimetres of patella and tibial tubercle must also be exposed for the bony harvest. The epitendineum is preserved so that it can be closed at the completion of the procedure (Fig. 1.160).

Mark the central one-third of the tendon with a marking pen and incise the tendon. The incision is made in line with the tendon fibres (Fig. 1.161).

Once both sides of the central third of the tendon have been incised, place an instrument behind the central portion and in front of the medial and lateral portions. Mark the bone the same width as the tendon. The bone plugs should be 2 cm in length (Fig. 1.162).

Mark the oscillating saw at a depth of 1 cm (Fig. 1.163).

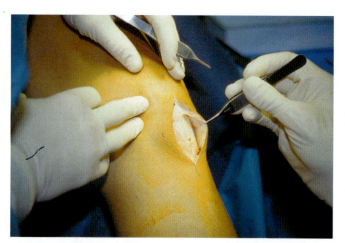

1.160

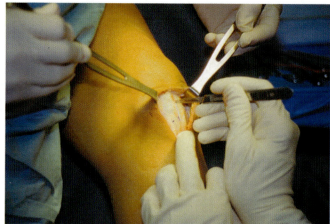

1.161

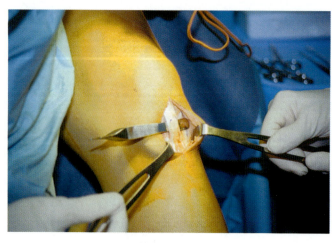

1.162

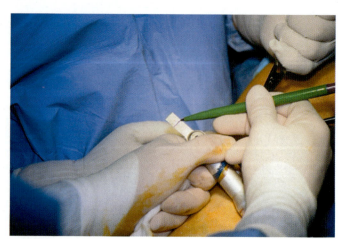

1.163

Harvest the tibial plug first to avoid any 'rundown' bleeding. Do not completely detach the tibial side at this time, as the continuity serves to maintain tension within the construct, which aids the creation of the patellar cuts (Fig. 1.164).

The patellar bone cuts are made at approximately a 45º angle. By bevelling the cuts the maximum width of bone plug is created with the minimum compromise to the patella. Avoid the use of a mallet in harvesting the patellar portion, as this will cause damage to the chondral surface. Cut the cortex with the small sagittal saw and attempt to taper the edges of the cuts to minimize the stress risers generated by the procedure (Fig. 1.165).

An osteotome can be used to pry or elevate the bone plug. The tibial bone plug can be cut deeper without concern for the articular surface. Leave a small amount of bone attached between the tibia and the graft until the very last. This permits harvesting of the patellar bone without the risk of dropping the graft (Fig. 1.166).

Once the central third of the patellar tendon has been harvested it can be taken to the back table to be prepared. The tendon defect will serve as the transpatellar tendon arthroscopy portal. The anteromedial portal can also be accessed through this skin incision by gentle medial skin retraction (Fig. 1.167).

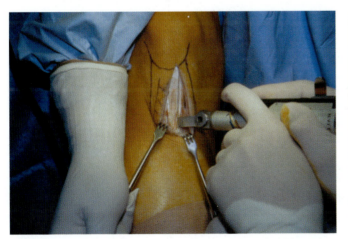

1.164

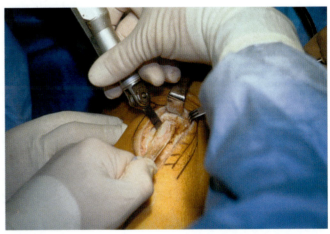

1.165

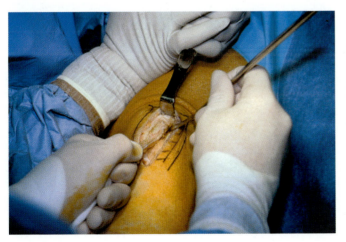

1.166

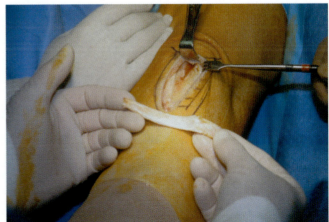

1.167

Curette out all sharp margins from the patellar plug graft site and obtain bone graft via the tibial plug graft site (Fig. 1.168).

Use a rongeur to remove excess bone as needed in order to slide the graft through the appropriate graft sizer. Any bone removed should be retained for grafting (Fig. 1.169a).

The graft must slide freely from one end of the sizer to the other. Provided that both slide through their respective sizing portals, the two ends may be different widths. The femoral plug must be of the same diameter or smaller than the tibial plug, as it will be passed via the tibial tunnel (Fig. 1.169b).

Prepare the graft by drilling two parallel holes in the bone plugs. This may be done free-hand or using a jig, as in this case (Fig. 1.170).

Pass a no. 5 Ethibond suture through each of the four drill holes. These will be used to pass the graft in the same way as is done with the soft tissue grafts. Once the femoral tunnel has been drilled the sutures passing through the femoral plug can be threaded through an Endobutton and tied (see Fig. 1.146). Cover the graft with a saline-soaked gauze until it is ready to be passed. The technique of preparation of the graft for insertion is described in the section on hamstring autograft preparation.

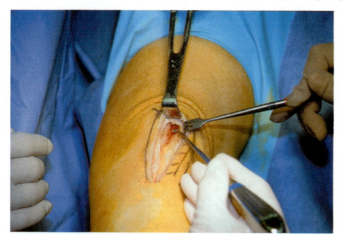

1.168

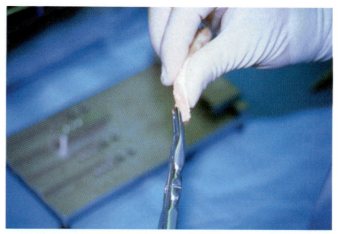

1.169a

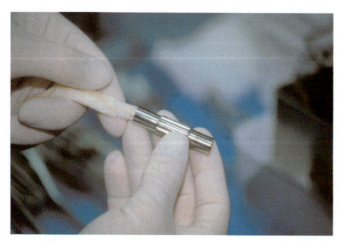

1.169b

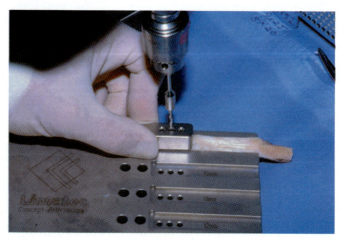

1.170

Notchplasty

Notchplasty is required to prevent impingement of the graft on the roof of the notch and on the medial wall of the lateral femoral condyle. Most arthroscopists will opt for a traditional notchplasty. Insert a gouge through an anteromedial portal and pass it across the intercondylar notch. Position the gouge at the superior aspect of the notch, planning to work laterally (Fig. 1.171).

Have the assistant tap the gouge into the chondral surface to its full depth with a mallet (Fig. 1.172).

Withdraw the gouge and move it inferiorly, leaving a small bridge between each fragment to facilitate removal with the grasper (Fig. 1.173).

Repeat the process until the inferior chondral surface has been reached. It is important to leave the fragments attached until they are ready to be removed (Fig. 1.174).

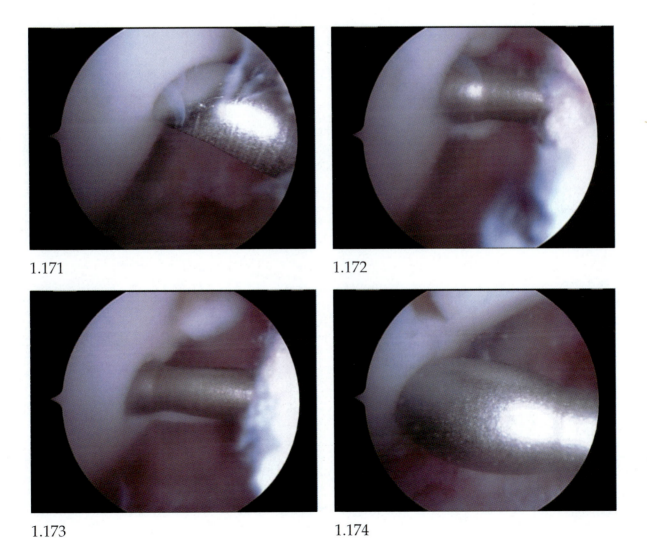

1.171

1.172

1.173

1.174

Once the anterior margin has been freed with the gouge, remove the fragments individually with a grasper (Fig. 1.175).

After all of the fragments have been removed, use a burr to smooth the anterior margin down to the level created by the gouge (Fig. 1.176).

Complete the notchplasty by working posteriorly with the burr until the posterior margin has been identified and it is possible to pass a probe around the posterior wall (Fig. 1.177).

Using this technique it can be difficult to remove the inferior chondral margin with a burr without damaging the tibial cartilage. A small curette can be used to remove this tissue (Fig. 1.178).

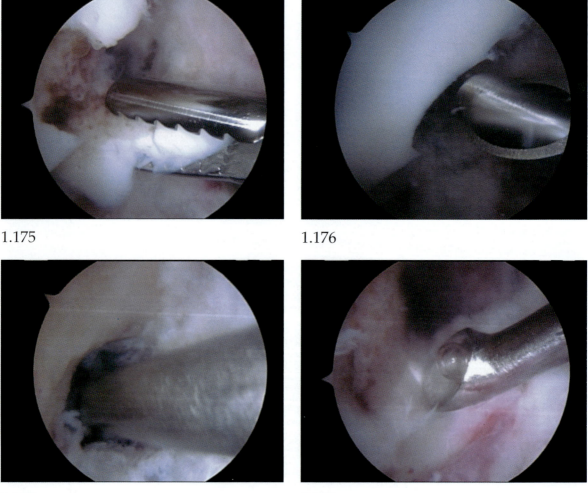

1.175

1.176

1.177

1.178

An alternative technique, which is quicker and more precise, is used by several of the surgeons at Orthopaedic Research of Virginia and Tuckahoe Orthopaedic Associates. Although the technique is in theory simple, it should only be attempted by experienced arthroscopists as there is a potential risk to the posterior neurovascular structures in the knee. This method removes the precise amount of notch and roof needed, regardless of whether the tibial tunnel is slightly more anterior or posterior.

Reintroduce the drill that was used to create the tibial tunnel back into the tunnel. Carefully push the drill bit through the tunnel and into the intercondylar notch (Fig. 1.179).

With the knee flexed the drill bit extends out of the tibia and into the intercondylar notch. With the drill running and under direct vision, gently flex and extend the knee. This will remove bone from the lateral aspect of the intercondylar notch which corresponds to the width of the drill bit and hence the width of the graft (Fig. 1.180).

The drill bit is shown here with the knee in full extension, and only a very small portion of the bit can be seen. The arthroscopic surgeon must be very careful as this procedure is performed because of the possible risk to the neurovascular structures in the posterolateral portion of the knee. This is because with the knee in full extension, the posterior structures of the knee are more tightly pressed against the posterior capsule (Fig. 1.181).

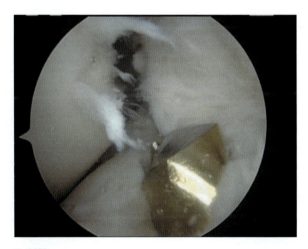

1.179

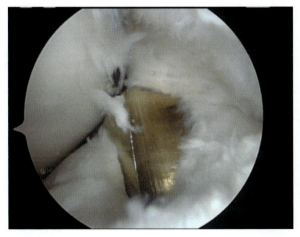

1.180

1.181

As the notchplasty is performed the surgeon may desire to drill a very small portion, retract the unturning drill bit into the tibial tunnel, flex the knee and check the progress of the notchplasty, before drilling completely across the femoral intercondylar notch (Fig. 1.182).

With the knee flexed, one can see that the notchplasty has been almost completely performed by the drill bit. With the knee in a flexed position and under direct view, gently flex and extend the knee. By pistoning the drill bit only a few centimetres a lateral wall notchplasty is achieved by the side-cutting edge of the drill bit (Fig. 1.183).

In this particular drill notchplasty the posteriormost portion of the notch has been left intact (Fig. 1.184).

The posterior cortex can be quickly removed with a burr. The posterolateral neurovascular structures have been protected by leaving this small portion of bone (Fig. 1.185).

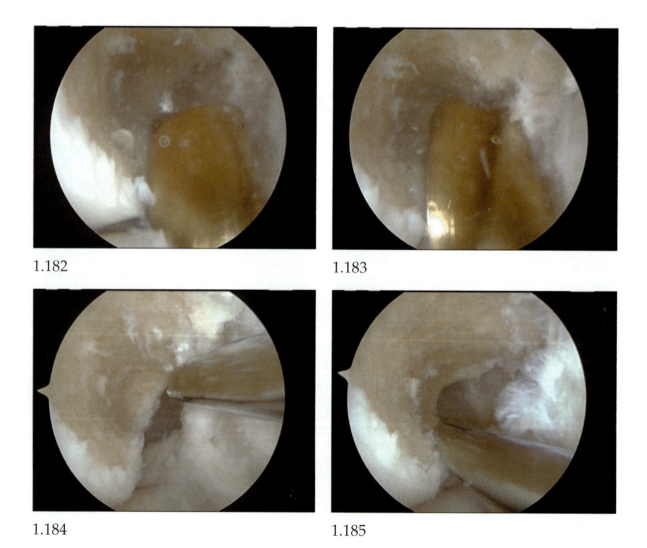

1.182

1.183

1.184

1.185

Tibial tunnel creation

Once the graft has been harvested and prepared attention should be turned to the tibial tunnel. The graft is usually introduced into the knee via the tibial tunnel and pulled through the intercondylar notch to exit via the femoral tunnel. It is therefore important to size the graft accurately using any of the commercially available sizing templates (see relevant sections on graft preparation) (Fig. 1.186).

The diameter of the tibial tunnel must allow for the passage of both ends of the graft. This is not usually a problem with hamstring or fascia lata grafts, as they are in uniform diameter. The patellar and tibial bone plugs of patellar tendon grafts are often different sizes. The smaller plug should be used for the femoral end and the larger for the tibial end. This allows a slightly smaller tunnel to be drilled on the femoral side.

To restore the biomechanics of the ACL as accurately as possible the tibial tunnel should be placed such that the exit is at the footprint of the original ACL, i.e. just in front of the posterior cruciate ligament (PCL) (Fig. 1.187).

Use a punch to start the excision of the ACL stump if this has not already been done. This is often faster than excising the whole ligament with a shaver (Fig. 1.188).

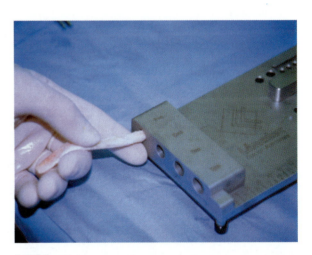

1.186

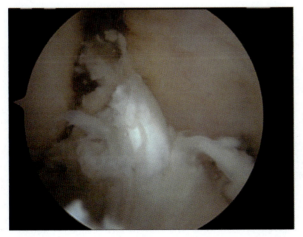

1.187

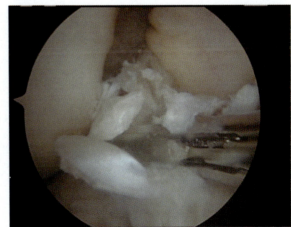

1.188

The excision can be completed with a shaver to expose the ACL footprint and the tibial spines. The better this is cleared, the easier the tunnel preparation will be (Fig. 1.189).

The tibial tunnel is drilled over a guide wire. Although it is theoretically possible to insert the wire freehand, most people will use a jig to simplify its accurate placement. There are a number of different jigs on the market (Fig. 1.190).

Insert the tip of the guide jig via the anteromedial portal. This allows easy access to the target site and positions the distal end on the medial side of the patellar tendon. The tip needs to be directed into the knee, and this requires a twisting movement to direct it round the medial femoral condyle (Fig. 1.191).

With the tip in approximately the correct position, the distal end should be placed at the site planned for the start of the tunnel. It is usually placed 1–2 cm medial to the patellar tendon, as this will give a straighter line of pull when the graft is being fed through into the tunnel (Fig. 1.192).

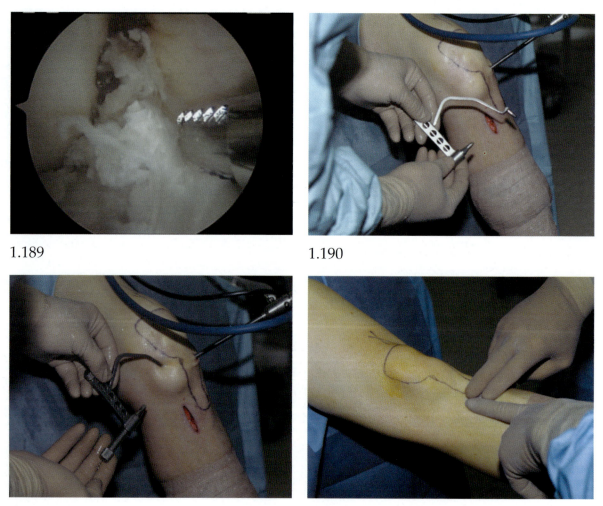

1.189

1.190

1.191

1.192

If a hamstring graft has been taken the incision that has already been made can be used for the tibial tunnel (Fig. 1.193).

If a patellar tendon or fascia lata graft is to be used an incision will have to be made, guided by the distal end of the jig. This only needs to be big enough to allow the graft to pass through (usually no more than 2 cm) (Fig. 1.194).

Once the skin incision has been made accurately position the tip of the jig so that the exit point of the guide wire will be through the ACL footprint. The precise position will vary from jig to jig (Fig. 1.195).

Place the distal end of the jig against the cortex of the tibia through the previously made skin incision and drill the wire through the tibia (Fig. 1.196).

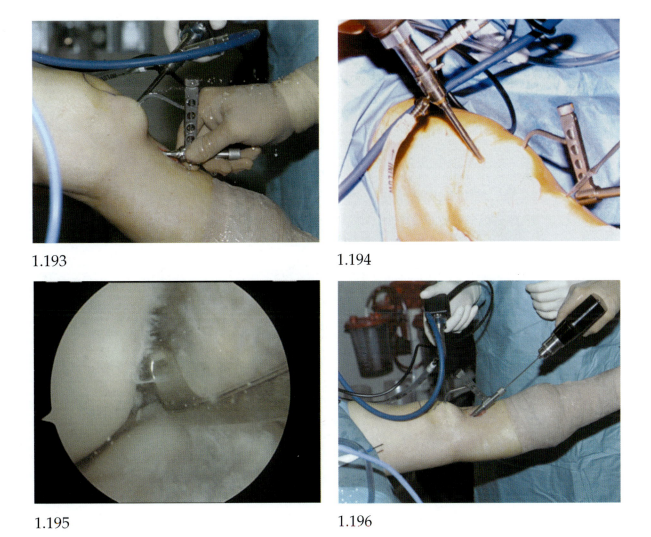

1.193

1.194

1.195

1.196

Once the tip of the wire can be seen in the joint, check that the position is correct and remove the jig. All of them have different methods of releasing from the wire, so practice beforehand (Fig. 1.197).

Make a final check that the wire is in the correct position before committing to drilling the tunnel (Fig. 1.198).

Place the selected tibial drill bit over the guide wire and drill through the cortex of the tibia (Fig. 1.199).

Watch the tip of the wire through the arthroscope throughout drilling to ensure that not only is the position correct but that the wire is not driven through the joint, as can sometimes happen (Fig. 1.200).

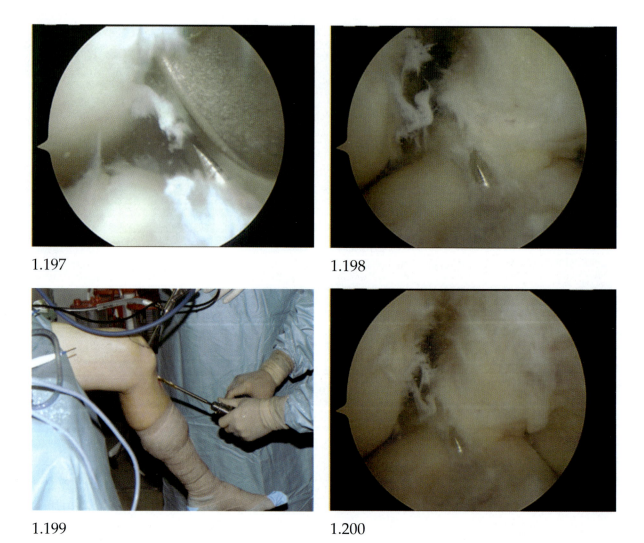

1.197

1.198

1.199

1.200

As soon as the drill bit appears in the joint the drill and wire can be removed (Fig. 1.201). Once the drill bit has been removed there is a large tunnel through which fluid can extravasate, which makes visualization difficult. Insert a plug into the tunnel to control this (Fig. 1.202).

A rim of articular cartilage will surround the intra-articular end of the tunnel. This reduces the effective diameter of the tunnel and can make passage of the graft difficult (Fig. 1.203).

Use a shaver to remove the loose articular cartilage and any bone debris from around the tibial tunnel (Fig. 1.204).

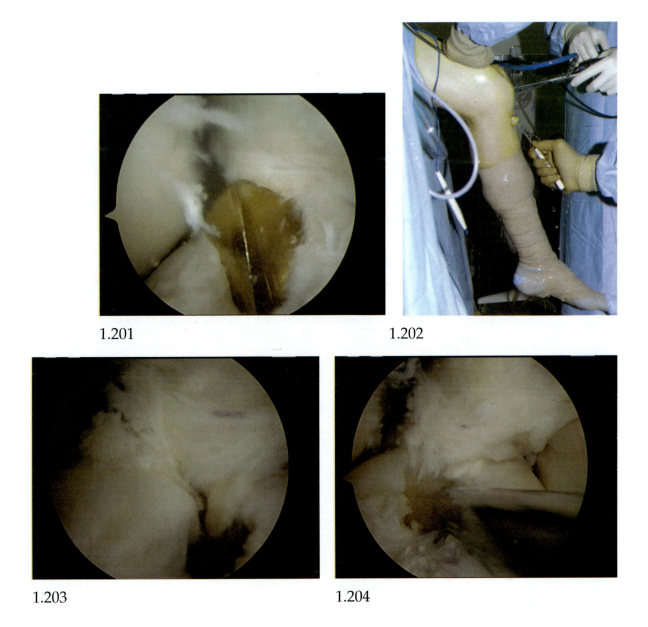

1.201

1.202

1.203

1.204

Inspect the tunnel rim and the tibial spine, as this may occasionally impinge on the graft once it has been passed. There is also often a posterior cartilage flap that needs to be removed (Fig. 1.205).

The tibial tunnel can now be used for the preparation of the femoral tunnel and passage of the graft, as described in the other sections (Fig. 1.206).

Femoral tunnel preparation

Once the tibial tunnel and the notchplasty have been performed a clear view of the tibial tunnel and the lateral wall of the intercondylar notch is obtained (Fig. 1.207).

Insert an intra-articular femoral aimer through the tibial tunnel. This device has a foot plate which is placed on the back cortex of the lateral femoral condyle. The distance from the foot plate to the centre of the pin is determined by the size of the graft. For example, if a 10 mm graft has been prepared then a 10 mm femoral aimer is chosen. This will place the centre of the femoral tunnel approximately 6 mm in front of the posterior cortex. Half of the diameter of the drill width is removed from each side of the pin. This leaves a 1 mm posterior bone bridge from the posterior edge of the femoral tunnel to the cortex (Fig. 1.208).

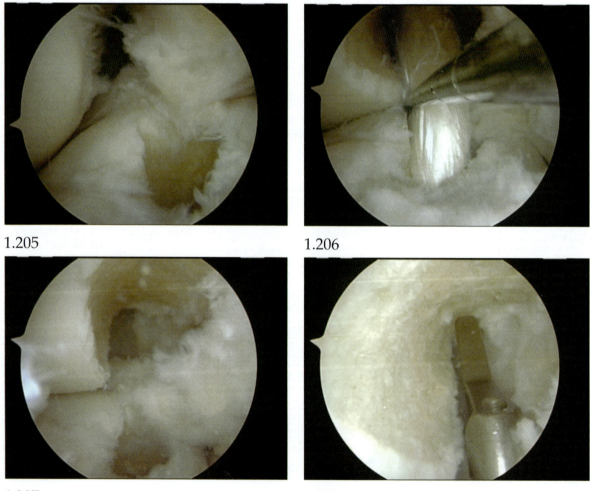

1.205

1.206

1.207

1.208

Once the foot plate is over the posterior cortex, insert a pin through the femoral aimer. Drill the pin into the femur far enough to make a pilot hole (Fig. 1.209).

Remove the pin and guide and assess the position of the pilot hole (Fig. 1.210).

Flex the knee maximally and, without reinserting the femoral aimer, reinsert the pin into the pilot hole. This enables the pin, and hence the femoral tunnel, to be directed more distally, making the exit point of the pin and the graft sutures more distal and easier to manage.

At this stage it is possible to reposition the guide pin, as shown here. Drill the pin through the lateral cortex. It does not need to be driven out through the skin (Fig. 1.211).

Once the guide pin is properly placed, insert the appropriate size of drill bit over it (Fig. 1.212).

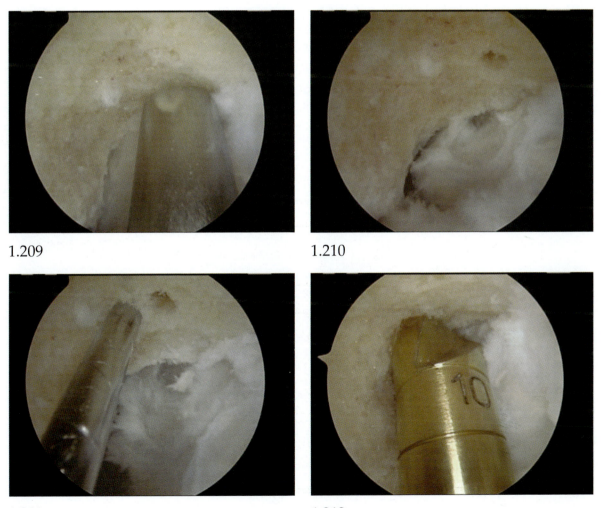

1.209

1.210

1.211

1.212

Two technical points at this juncture: first, the edge of the drill bit should be touching the PCL. The aim is to re-establish the cruciate relationship of the PCL and the ACL, therefore the medialmost portion of the soon-to-be implanted ACL graft should be in contact with the PCL. Second, the preferred graft position is at approximately the 11 o'clock position in a right knee and in the 1 o'clock position in a left knee.

With the guide pin correctly positioned, overdrill to a depth of 3–4 cm. To use the Endobutton for fixation it is mandatory that the large drill bit does not breach the femoral cortex. If it does compromise the femoral cortex, then Endobutton fixation is no longer possible (Fig. 1.213).

A view of the femoral tunnel with the arthroscope through the transpatellar tendon portal is illustrated (Fig. 1.214). Through this view, the femoral tunnel and the completeness of the bone tunnel can be adequately evaluated. If you occasionally see the tunnel with a small amount of periosteum at the articular end this is not a concern. Cortex must be present at the proximal end of the tunnel, and bone should encircle the vast majority of the tunnel.

For the Endobutton to pass, the channel through the lateral femoral cortex created by the guide pin must be enlarged. The 4.5 mm drill bit will broach the cortex to allow the Endobutton to pass out of the lateral femoral cortex. Illustrated is the small-diameter drill bit sliding over the guide pin (Fig. 1.215).

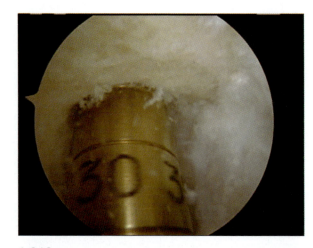

1.213

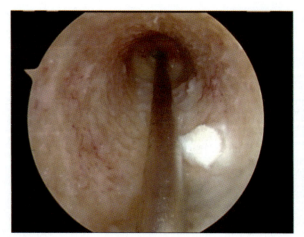

1.214

1.215

Measure the total length of the femoral tunnel. The tunnel can be deepened to minimize any difficulty in passing the graft or seating the Endobutton. A minimum of 2 cm of graft must be placed into the tunnel (Fig. 1.216).

Calculate the length of the Endobutton loop to be used as follows: the length of the loop must equal the difference between the lengths of the large and small tunnels and allow 6 mm for the Endobutton to toggle.

Example: If the depth to the cortex is 60 mm and the large tunnel has been drilled to 40 mm, the Endobutton loop must be a minimum of 20 mm to allow the button to reach the lateral cortex. A further 6 mm must be allowed for the button to toggle. In this instance a 30 mm loop should be used. Once the Endobutton is in place the graft will end 30 mm from the lateral cortex. In this case, with a 60 mm total depth, 30 mm of graft will remain in the tunnel, which is adequate.

Use a shaver to smooth the edges of the femoral tunnel. This instrument is less aggressive than the burr and will produce a smooth edge (Fig. 1.217).

Reinspect the femoral tunnel to ensure that the lateral femoral cortex is intact (Fig. 1.218).

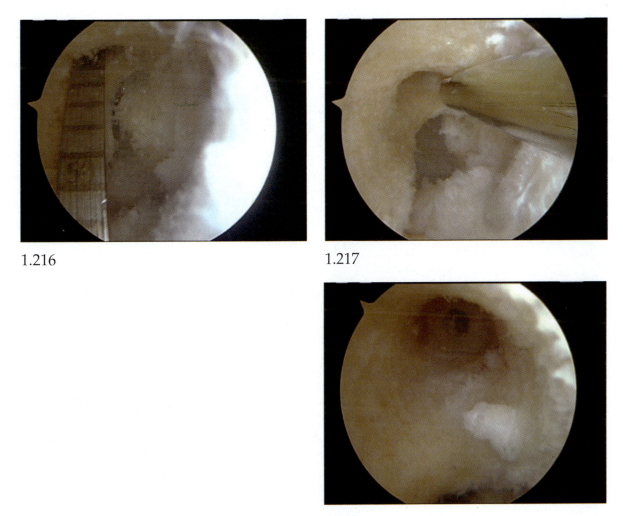

1.216

1.217

1.218

Passing the graft

Pass a long pin with an eyelet from the tibial tunnel through the femoral tunnel to exit through the anterolateral portion of the thigh (Fig. 1.219).

Pass a suture through the eyelet and tie it in a loop. Pass the two Ethibond guide sutures from the Endobutton through the loop. Pull the suture loop out through the anterolateral thigh. To ease the passage of the loop the knot should be placed close to the eyelet (Fig. 1.220).

Remove the guide pin from the anterolateral thigh, drawing the suture loop with it (Fig. 1.221).

By pulling on the sutures draw the graft into the joint via the tibial tunnel (Fig. 1.222).

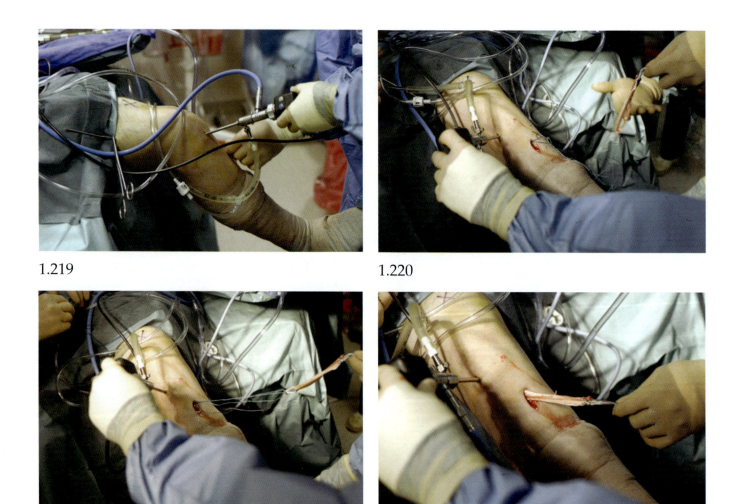

1.219

1.220

1.221

1.222

Use the suture loop to draw the Endobutton sutures through the femoral tunnel and the skin. The Endobutton is just about ready to pass into the femoral tunnel (Fig. 1.223).

Apply tension to one of the Endobutton sutures. The Endobutton will flip into an elongated position and will pass through the femoral tunnel (Fig. 1.224).

Once the second mark on the graft passes into the femoral tunnel the Endobutton is clear of the femoral cortex. Apply tension to both sutures. The Endobutton will 'flip' and come to lie flat against the femoral cortex. The small size of the drill hole in the lateral femoral cortex will not allow the flattened Endobutton back into the lateral femoral cortical hole.

It is important to ensure that the length of the Endobutton loop is sufficient to allow the 6 mm clearance of the Endobutton outside the femur to allow it to flip. If the loop is too short and the graft is against the end of the tunnel, the button will not flip.

The Endobutton can be 'toggled' outside the lateral femoral cortex. This toggling is a key confirming that the Endobutton has exited the femoral cortex and is sitting outside the femur instead of in the tunnel. By alternating pulls on the guide sutures, one can be confident that the Endobutton is extraosseous. If there is any question in your mind about the position of the Endobutton, then we suggest several options. Pull on the graft from the tibial tunnel, and

if indeed it is not outside the femoral cortex it will pull back into the knee joint. You may also check the position with either X-ray or fluoroscopy to ensure that the Endobutton is sitting on the lateral femoral cortex.

With the graft in place its vertical orientation should be observed. Here it does touch the PCL and there is adequate notchplasty to prevent impingement from the lateral femoral cortex. Look up at the roof of the notchplasty to assure that there are no osteophytes at the entry into the femoral tunnel (Fig. 1.225).

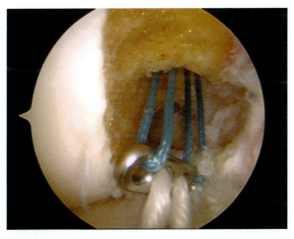

1.223

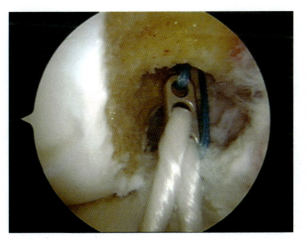

1.224

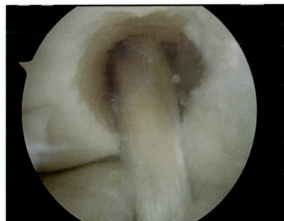

1.225

Inspect the inferior margin of the lateral wall, as this is often a site of impingement (Fig. 1.226).

With the knee in full extension, view the graft very carefully to assure that it does 'tuck' under the roof of the notch and is not impinged. You should also watch the graft closely at the exit of the tibial tunnel to ensure that as you bring the knee into full extension, the graft is not pulled back into the knee joint because of roof impingement. Once you are sure that you have an adequate notchplasty, then you may proceed to the next step and the arthroscopic instruments are removed (Fig. 1.227).

Graft tensioning and fixation

The allograft is tensioned with a device placed on the foot like a boot and wrapped to the leg with a sterile bandage. This will allow a greater amount of tension to be placed on the graft than can be provided by manual distraction (Fig. 1.228).

The tensioning boot has left and right knee options, and this should first be dialled in. Pass the suture ends round the stud on the wheel and tie them securely. To prevent slippage two needle holders can be used as clamps across the sutures (Fig. 1.229).

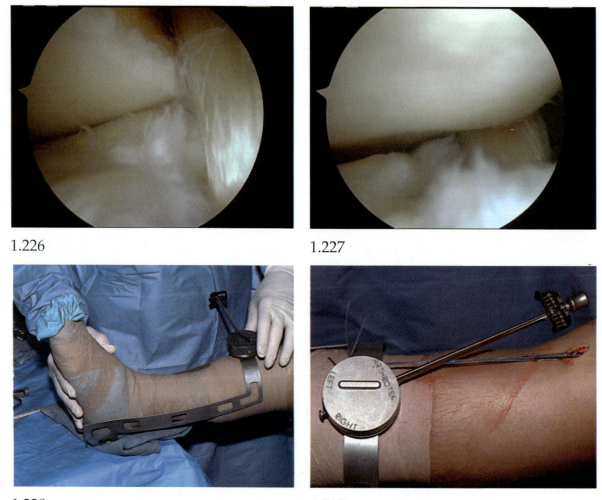

1.226

1.227

1.228

1.229

Dial the torque tensioner to 20 lb tension (Fig. 1.230).

Cycle the knee 0–90º 10 times to take up the slack in the graft. Retension the boot to 20 lb (Fig. 1.231).

Graft tibial fixation is performed using an interference screw. There are a variety of screw types available, both metal and bioabsorbable. The decision is up to the individual surgeon (Fig. 1.232).

Pass a fine guide wire through the tibial tunnel alongside the graft. Check the wire's position using the arthroscope. The wire will rotate as the screw is inserted. It is therefore desirable to place the wire on the left side of the graft to allow for clockwise rotation (Fig. 1.233).

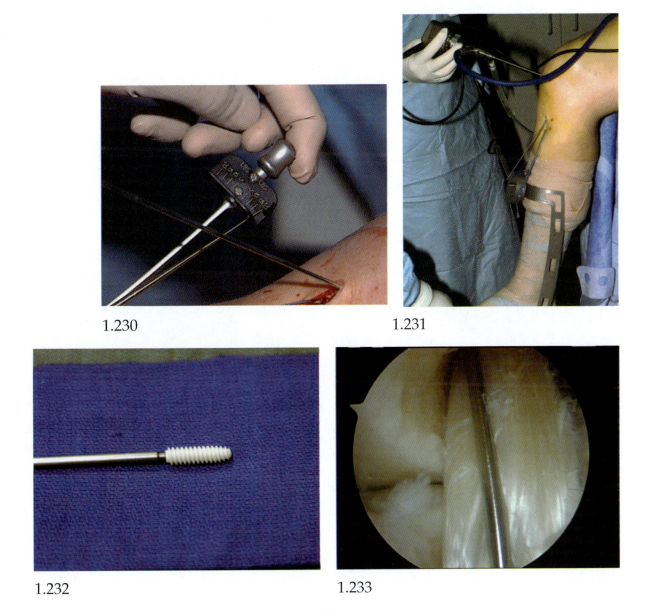

1.230

1.231

1.232

1.233

Insert the screw using the cannulated screwdriver. Follow the progress of the screw arthroscopically to confirm that it does not impinge on the joint (Fig. 1.234).

Once the screw is in position, remove the wire. Examine the graft using a probe to confirm that the tension is appropriate and the fixation secure (Fig. 1.235).

Supplemental fixation can be used if desired. We use either three staples inserted using an air-powered 'Stapilizer' gun or a screw/post system (Fig. 1.236).

Using the stapilizer, insert three staples across the distal graft. Press down firmly and allow the 'hammer' to drive each staple two to three times to ensure that the grip on the graft is secure (Fig. 1.237).

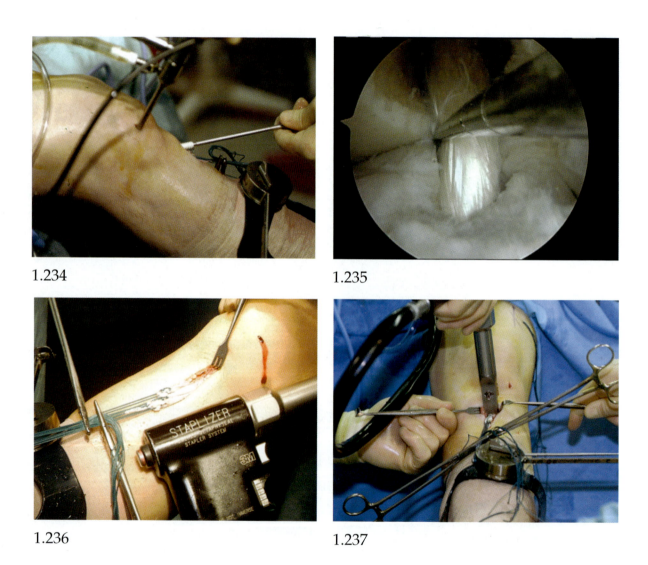

1.234

1.235

1.236

1.237

Inspect the staples to ensure that they are secure. The tensioning boot can then be removed and excess graft and suture material excised (Fig. 1.238).

If there is enough graft protruding from the tibial tunnel a ligament screw and washer can be used as supplemental fixation (Fig. 1.239).

Pull the graft ends to one side and, using a 4.5 mm bit, drill a hole through the anterior cortex behind the graft (Fig. 1.240).

Tap the hole and spread the ends of the graft. Insert the screw and washer through the space so that the washer traps the graft. When it is secure, remove the tensioning boot and excise any excess graft and suture material (Fig. 1.241).

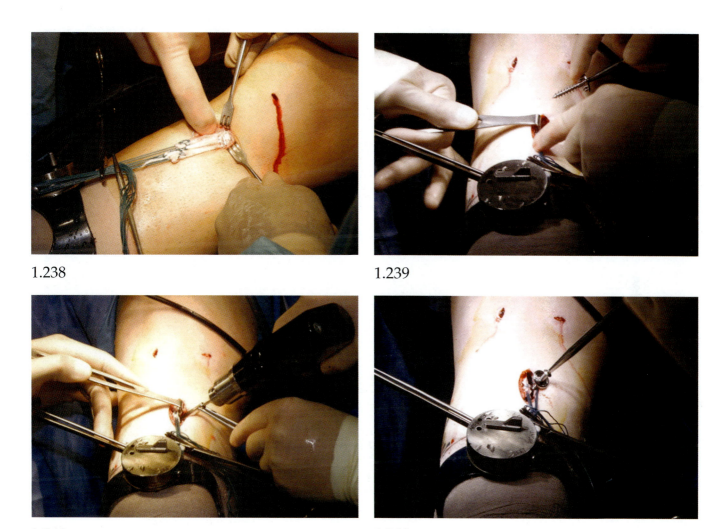

1.238

1.239

1.240

1.241

2 SHOULDER ARTHROSCOPY

INTRODUCTION

The shoulder is far less frequently arthroscoped than the knee and requires significantly more experience before meaningful surgery can be performed.

In this chapter we describe and illustrate a number of aspects of shoulder arthroscopy, from patient setup to rotator cuff repair. The 'mini-open' rotator cuff repair is also included, as many surgeons will not perform totally arthroscopic repairs or will use this technique while they are learning the arthroscopic technique.

There are many ways of doing all of the things described in this chapter and we do not claim that ours is the only way. We have, however, found that the techniques described here are reproducible, safe, and facilitate good arthroscopic surgery. Not everyone will want to use the traction device we illustrate; however, all surgeons should perform an examination under anaesthetic prior to arthroscopy. Likewise, many surgeons will prefer to orientate the camera differently (making the glenoid vertical, for example), but the principle of a routine and systematic examination of the whole joint must remain the same.

All of the procedures described are in the lateral position. Many surgeons prefer the 'beach chair' position and there is no contraindication to performing any of the procedures using this alternative setup. It has been our experience, however, that some of the procedures are more difficult in the recumbent position, and we therefore perform all surgery in the lateral position.

Our hope is that surgeons reading this chapter will combine the information we present with their own experience and preferences. Only this way will arthroscopy progress and develop.

Complications and pitfalls

Shoulder arthroscopy is technically more complex than knee arthroscopy. The setup and positioning of the patient are far more crucial and joint access is more difficult.

The patient position and setup are outlined in the relevant section, and it is important that the operating surgeon be present to supervise: if the patient is not tilted back 20–30º access via the anterior portal can be very difficult, particularly in larger patients. It is also critical to check that bony prominences and nerves are adequately padded. This includes the contralateral brachial plexus and ulnar nerve, as well as both knees and ankles.

A fluid pump is essential for shoulder arthroscopy to control bleeding. It is the surgeon's responsibility to check that the pump pressure is appropriate. There are a number of different types of pump available and each has a recommended pressure for shoulder arthroscopy. If the pressure falls too low the joint or bursa will fill with blood, and if it is too high the soft tissues will fill with fluid, making surgery more difficult. It is also important to ensure that the fluid reservoir bag does not run out, as this will have the same end result of the joint being obscured with blood. Once bleeding starts it is difficult to control.

Neurovascular risks

The brachial plexus lies in close proximity to the shoulder and all surgeons must be aware of the relevant anatomy. The anterior portal lies close to the musculocutaneous nerve as it enters the undersurface of the conjoint tendon. A low anterior portal, which has not been described here but is used by some surgeons for Bankart repair, can place the axillary nerve at risk as it runs under the inferior border of the subscapularis. The axillary nerve may also be damaged during inferior capsular procedures. As long as any sutures and capsular releases are performed close to the glenoid neck the nerve is relatively safe. It is advised, however, that diathermy not be used for the inferiormost portion of a capsular release.

The posterior portal can potentially damage the suprascapular nerve and associated vessels as they cross the posterior glenoid neck, although this is rarely seen in practice. The same structures are at risk during the transglenoid capsular repair if the guide pin is placed too laterally.

Traction may also cause neurological problems if not used correctly. Excessive traction may damage both the median and the ulnar nerves. Fortunately this is usually only a neuropraxia, which resolves quickly. If the traction device is applied too tightly to the forearm a neuropraxia of the superficial branch of the radial nerve can occur which can be troublesome but will resolve eventually.

Attention should also be paid to the contralateral side of the body to prevent neurological damage. To this end the axilla, the lateral aspect of the knee and the ankle should be padded. The elbow should also be inspected to ensure that the ulnar nerve is not being compressed.

PATIENT SETUP

The preparation of the patient for arthroscopy of the shoulder is far more complex than for the knee. If it is not done correctly, not only is the surgery more difficult but also harm may come to the patient. It is essential that the operating surgeon be present throughout the procedure.

In our practice the use of an interscalene block is routine, and the authors would recommend this to all surgeons. It is far easier to have the block inserted after the induction of anaesthesia but before surgery, as the anatomical landmarks will become distorted later.

By placing the patient in 20–30º of posterior tilt, not only is the glenoid parallel to the floor but access via the anterior portal is facilitated. If the patient is very large this tilt may need to be increased to allow full movement of the instruments. Once the patient is in position it is advisable to pad the head lightly and secure it: the anaesthetist often requests this step. Ensure that there is adequate padding of all prominences and nerves, as shoulder arthroscopy can take a long time.

Attention to the arrangement of the operating room can make a significant difference to the ease of surgery. Ensure that both the surgeon and the assistant can see the monitors clearly, and that the scrub nurse is in such a position that instruments can be handed to the surgeon without anyone having to twist or turn.

In our practice the surgeon stands behind the patient and both face the monitor. The assistant stands at the head and the nurse to the foot end of the surgeon. This arrangement can make it difficult for the assistant to see the monitor clearly at times, and means that they are often operating 'upside-down'. An alternative is to have the assistant facing the surgeon, but this can obscure the surgeon's view of the monitor and means that the assistant needs a second monitor behind the surgeon. Either this, or both share a monitor at the patient's head and both have to twist, with the surgeon's back to the scrub nurse. Experience, local circumstances and personal preference will make the final decision, but it is worth experimenting with the alternatives.

When the patient's skin is prepared it is important to extend the prepared area up the neck as far as possible, distally to the elbow, anteriorly to at least the nipple line, and posteriorly to the medial border of the scapula. Again, this allows for unrestricted access to the joint. Ensure that the distal arm is wrapped securely as the traction tends to pull the wrapping off. Resist the temptation to wrap very tightly, as neurapraxia of the superficial radial nerve has been experienced.

Place the patient initially in the supine position on the operating table for induction of general anaesthesia. An interscalene block is preferred for supplementary analgesia, and this is performed at this time (Fig. 2.1).

Roll the patient into the lateral position with the beanbag in place; 20–30º posterior tilt facilitates access to the anterior portal (Fig. 2.2).

Protect the brachial plexus with an axillary roll. Use pillows to protect the peroneal nerve of the downside leg and to prevent pressure between the legs.

Once the patient is placed in the lateral position, use tape to secure their pelvis to the bed to prevent rolling (Fig. 2.3).

Pad the head lightly. It may also be taped for stabilization. Excessive padding can cause access problems when using instruments later in the procedure (Fig. 2.4).

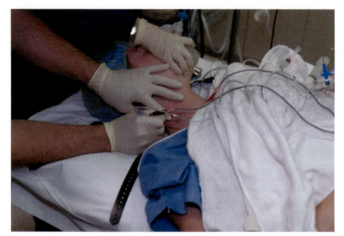

2.1

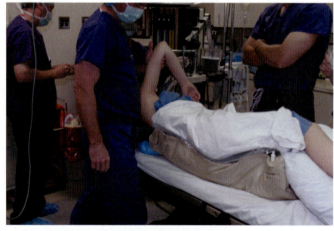

2.2

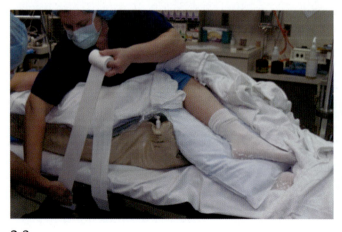

2.3

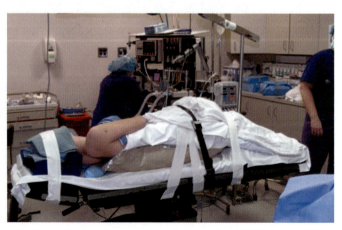

2.4

An important part of the surgical procedure is the examination under anaesthesia. By allowing the weight of the arm to load the shoulder the stability of the shoulder is tested, as is the range of motion. Anterior–posterior and inferior tension is placed on the humeral head. Note the amount and direction of the laxity or instability (Fig. 2.5).

Scrub the patient and paint with an iodine solution. This should extend below the elbow and allow access to both the front and the back of the shoulder (Fig. 2.6).

Quarter the shoulder with surgical towels to square the surgical field (Fig. 2.7).

Place a plastic U-drape around the arm, with the tails projected towards the head (Fig. 2.8).

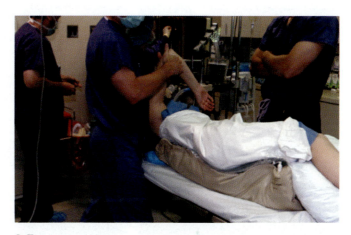

2.5

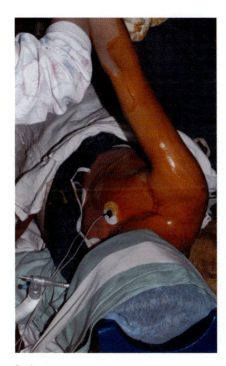

2.6

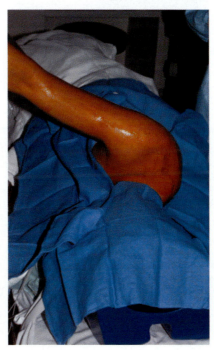

2.7

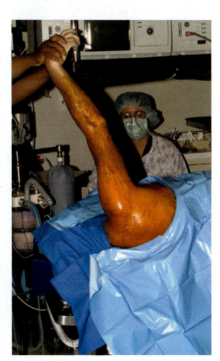

2.8

The arm traction device is an impervious sleeve which is placed over the unsterile hand and up the arm. Wrap a sterile bandage snugly around the sleeved extremity to prevent the traction sleeve from being pulled off during the procedure. The bandage should extend proximal to the end of the traction sleeve to seal it, as the hand is not prepared and is thus not sterile (Fig. 2.9).

Place an extremity drape over the shoulder to provide a complete sterile field. At the superior posterior margin of the shoulder, occasionally the elastic portion of the extremity drape will need to be cut to allow it to be placed more completely around the shoulder (Fig. 2.10).

Once the sterile field has been established, place the arm in traction: 15 lb is generally used for an average-size male patient. This should be evaluated carefully for patients who are smaller. This shoulder traction device is placed at the foot of the bed opposite the shoulder that is being operated on. With the patient in the lateral position this is the side of the table that the patient is facing (Fig. 2.11).

Draw the anatomical landmarks on the skin after the application of traction. These are the coracoid, clavicle, acromioclavicular joint (ACJ), acromion and scapular spine. As the shoulder becomes engorged during surgery the landmarks will move, and for this reason some surgeons prefer not to use them (Fig. 2.12).

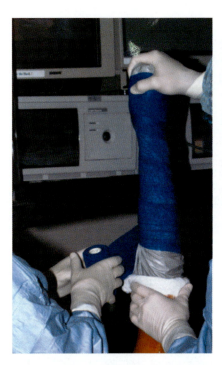

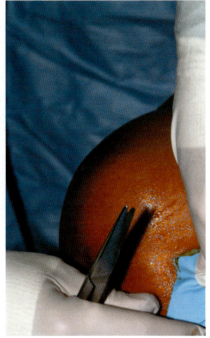

2.9

2.10

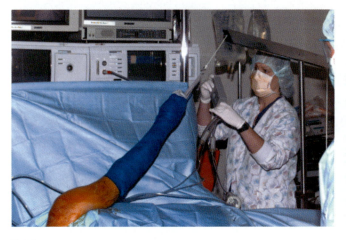

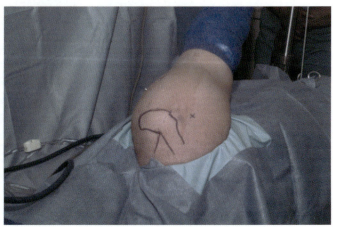

2.11

2.12

PORTAL CREATION

As with the knee, careful portal placement can mean the difference between a smooth, trouble-free arthroscopic procedure and one which is beset with difficulty in access and instrument manipulation. The temptation with the posterior portal is to make it too lateral and too high. It must be remembered that the lateral edge of the acromion is roughly at the level of the greater tuberosity, and that the articular surface is medial to this. As the joint and soft tissues distend the portal will rise, making visualization of the anteroinferior joint difficult. The anterior, rotator interval portal should be made quickly, before the joint swells. This applies in particular with the large patient, where it may be difficult to drive the trocar all the way to the skin. If this happens a Wissinger rod or a switching stick may be helpful. Take care when positioning the anterior portal. The rotator interval is a neurovascular 'safe zone'. If the portal is made lower, into the subscapularis, the musculocutaneous nerve is at risk. If the trocar is aimed too medially (toward the coracoid) the axillary nerve and the brachial plexus are compromised.

To obtain access to the subacromial bursa it is advisable to withdraw the trocar almost completely from the deltoid. This simple step gives a better angle of approach and makes it easier to move the arthroscope within the bursa. Using a spinal needle to identify the correct position for the lateral portal ensures that not only will the portal allow access to the bursa, but that the relevant structures within the bursa can be reached. On occasion, if there is dense tissue within the bursa it may not be possible to see the needle. In these cases aim the needle at the arthroscope and 'walk' it down to the tip, where it should be possible to see it.

We do not routinely make any of the 'alternative' portals, e.g. the posterolateral, as we have found those described here to be sufficient. There are occasions when further portals have to be created, for example during surgery for anterior instability, and the surgeon should not hesitate to do so if the procedure requires them. If the original portal is not providing adequate access (either because of incorrect placement or for other reasons) there is no point in struggling on, as this will not benefit either the patient or the surgeon. Create a better portal and finish the operation.

The bony landmarks have been included in this picture for clarity. The skin marks will move as the shoulder swells (Fig. 2.13).

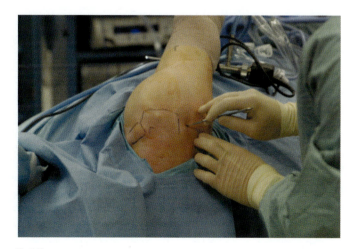

2.13

To provide a reference which is based on each patient and not on an arbitrary distance we place two to three fingers on the lateral border of the acromion and the thumb on its posterior margin. The incision is thus made at the intersection of these two lines, just beneath the thumb (Fig. 2.14).

Place the arthroscope sheath and blunt trocar into the incision. With the trocar tip, palpate the interval between the glenoid and the humeral head. Push the trocar through the posterior capsule, aiming towards the coracoid process anteriorly (Fig. 2.15).

Place the arthroscope into the sheath and confirm the intra-articular placement of the arthroscope. Once this quick evaluation is performed an anterior portal can be created (Fig. 2.16).

Identify the interval between the biceps tendon, the subscapularis and the glenoid (the rotator cuff interval). Push the arthroscope forward into this space (Fig. 2.17).

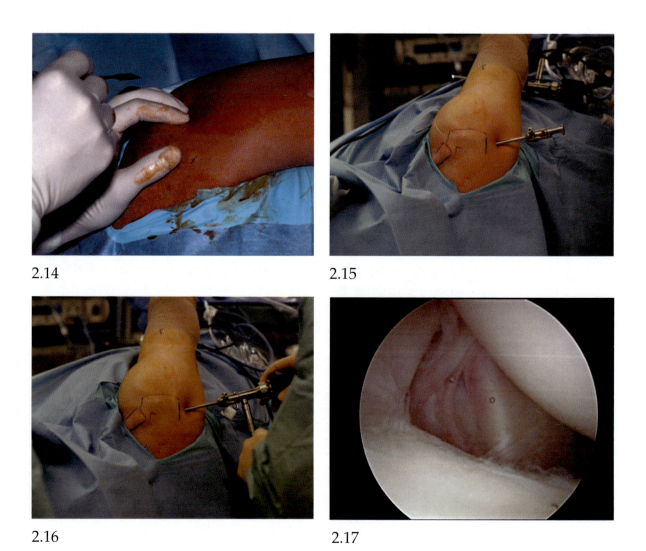

2.14

2.15

2.16

2.17

Reinsert the blunt trocar into the arthroscope sheath. Push this through the anterior capsule until it is palpable under the anterior skin (Fig. 2.18).

With the sheath tenting the skin, make a small anterior incision and push the blunt trocar through (Fig. 2.19).

Remove the trocar from a small plastic cannula 4.5 × 76 mm and place the cannula over the tip of the trocar. This will allow the blue cannula to be pushed back into the shoulder (Fig. 2.20).

The plastic cannula now sits inside the glenohumeral joint and the arthroscope is replaced into its sheath. The blue cannula can then be visualized within the joint (Fig. 2.21).

To create a portal for inspection of the subacromial bursa the same posterior portal incision is used. Remove arthroscope from the sleeve and reintroduce the blunt trocar.

Withdraw the sleeve and trocar until the tip is outside the joint capsule but not out of the deltoid muscle.

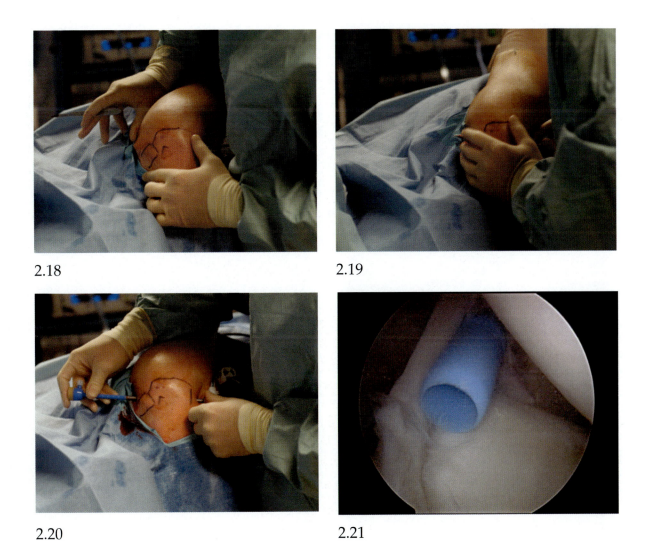

2.18

2.19

2.20

2.21

Reintroduce the instrument, aiming at the undersurface of the acromion lateral to the ACJ (Fig. 2.22).

Sweep the tip of the trocar medial to lateral to clear the bursa. The undersurface of the acromion should be felt with the tip of the trocar if it is positioned correctly.

Remove the trocar and reintroduce the arthroscope (Fig. 2.23).

With the arthroscope in the subacromial bursa, from the posterior portal turn the light source to view the undersurface of the acromion. We prefer to maintain an anatomical orientation, therefore with the patient on their side the cuff is to the right and the acromion to the left (Fig. 2.24).

To create a lateral working portal for the subacromial bursa, mark an entry point on the skin one-third of the way back from the anterior edge of the acromion and three fingers' breadth down the arm (Fig. 2.25).

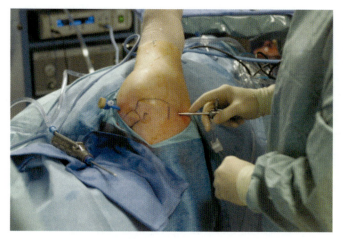

2.22

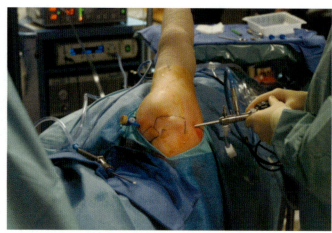

2.23

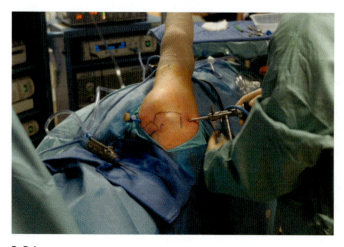

2.24

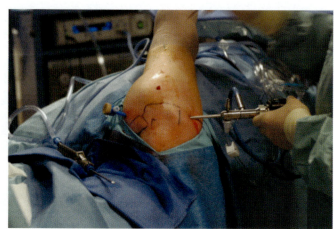

2.25

Introduce an 18 g spinal needle from this point, aiming at the tip of the arthroscope (Fig. 2.26).

If there is dense bursal tissue and a poor view it may be necessary to aim the needle at the scope itself and 'walk' it down to the tip by touch alone.

With a no. 11 blade make an incision over the spinal needle and introduce a 4.5 mm blue cannula (Fig. 2.27).

Again, if the bursal tissue is dense it may be easier to introduce a shaver. The bursal tissue can then be removed (Fig. 2.28).

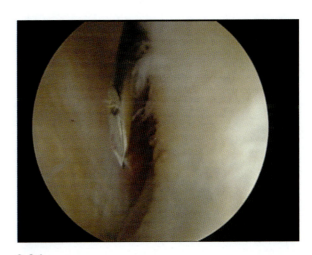

2.26

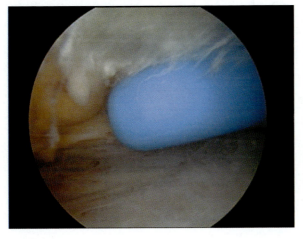

2.27

2.28

86

NORMAL GLENOHUMERAL ARTHROSCOPY

Arthroscopically, the shoulder joint has two compartments, the glenohumeral joint and the subacromial bursa. In contrast to the knee, where a normal joint should probably never be seen, the glenohumeral joint may be normal if all the pathology is located superior to the rotator cuff. As with the knee it is important to have a routine to ensure that no pathology is missed. It is helpful to have an assistant who can elevate the humeral head to improve access to the anteroinferior structures and abduct the arm if the insertion of the rotator cuff cannot be seen.

It may be necessary to use the shaver early on in the examination if there is synovium obscuring the view. Once the arthroscope has been removed from the joint there will be bleeding, and reinspection becomes very difficult.

Again, as with the knee, the experienced arthroscopist may deviate slightly from the routine examination to inspect the area of suspected pathology first. This enables the scrub nurse and circulating staff to prepare any equipment that may be needed while the rest of the systematic examination is being completed.

The patient is placed on the operating table as previously described. Make a posterior portal using the landmarks described and introduce the arthroscope, directing it at the coracoid (Fig. 2.29).

Once the arthroscope is in the joint orientate it so that the glenoid face lies horizontally at the bottom of the image. This orientation should be maintained throughout the procedure, and is done by keeping the camera in a fixed orientation and only rotating the light source to alter the view.

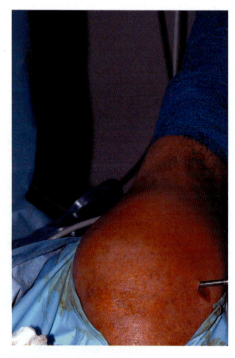

2.29

The humeral head is to the top right of the image and the glenoid face lies inferiorly. The biceps can be seen coming off the superior glenoid labrum and running up over the humeral head. The subscapularis can be seen running vertically behind the humeral head and the glenoid.

Identify the long head of biceps, glenoid, humeral head, subscapularis and the rotator interval. These are the landmarks of the glenohumeral joint. Inspect subscapularis at this stage, as the view can become obscured once the cannula is in situ (Fig. 2.30).

Drive the arthroscope into the rotator interval, aiming just above the free border of the subscapularis (Fig. 2.31).

Exchange the arthroscope for the blunt trocar, keeping some forward pressure at this point to ensure that the position is not lost (Fig. 2.32).

Push the trocar through the anterior capsule until the skin is tented (Fig. 2.33).

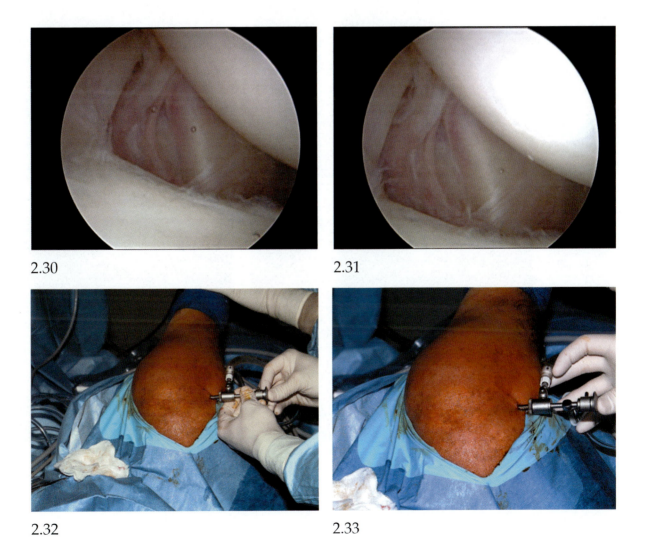

2.30

2.31

2.32

2.33

Make a skin incision over the trocar tip. It is often helpful to have an assistant do this while the surgeon maintains pressure (Fig. 2.34).

Railroad a blue 4.5 mm cannula into the joint over the trocar tip. Keep the sheath firmly against the cannula (Fig. 2.35).

Exchange the trocar for the arthroscope, again continuing the contact between the two instruments. This helps if the cannula has not been completely inserted into the joint. All that is required is for simple advancement using the trocar as a guide. If the trocar has been removed this is a far more complex step (Fig. 2.36).

Inspect the biceps insertion and assess for a possible superior labral anterior posterior tear (SLAP); use the probe to lift the insertion off the glenoid and to palpate the biceps origin (Fig. 2.37).

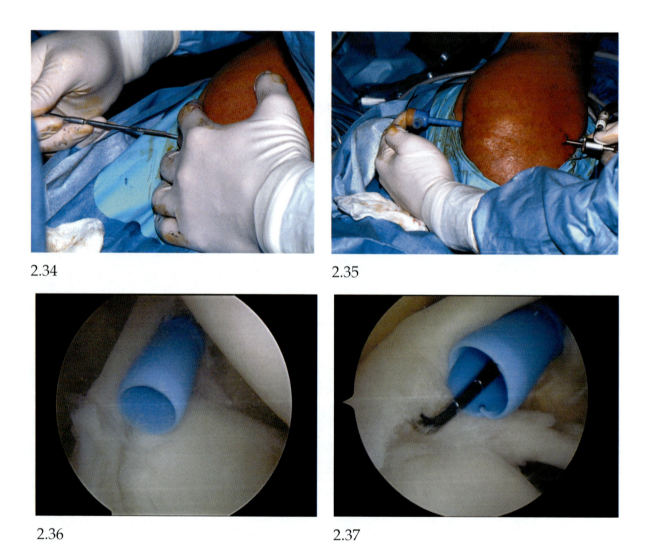

2.34

2.35

2.36

2.37

Inspect the biceps tendon and follow it up over the humeral head. The tendon needs to be assessed for appearance and quality (Fig. 2.38).

Rotate the light source to inspect the undersurface of the rotator cuff and the cuff insertion. As the posterior border of the bicipital groove is the anterior border of supraspinatus it is a simple move to see this (Fig. 2.39).

Position the blue cannula above the biceps tendon to enable palpation of the cuff with the probe (Fig. 2.40).

If there is significant synovitis or fraying of the rotator cuff it may be necessary to debride this with the shaver to improve the view (Fig. 2.41).

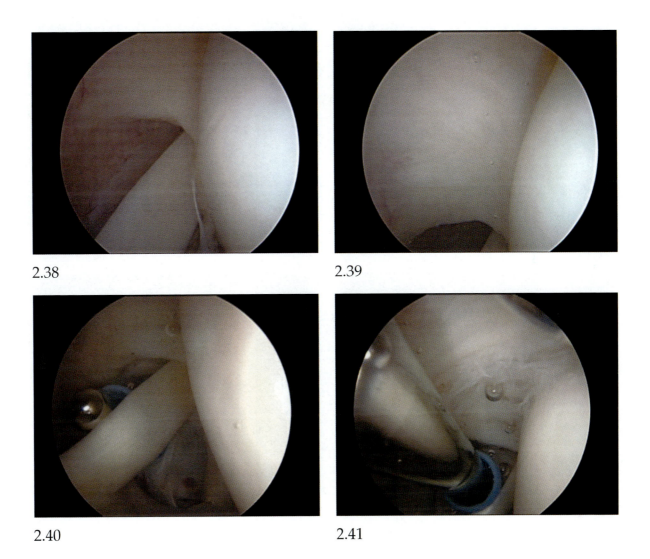

2.38

2.39

2.40

2.41

The insertion of the rotator cuff can then be followed posteriorly by rotating the light source and withdrawing the arthroscope. At this stage it may help to have an assistant abduct the shoulder slightly (Fig. 2.42).

At the posterior aspect of the humeral head the bare area can be seen to start with a normal cuff insertion (Fig. 2.43).

Inspect the bare area and distinguish it from a broca lesion (Fig. 2.44).

In some patients it will be possible to inspect the insertion of infraspinatus into the posterior aspect of the humerus. In many there will be some synovitis, which obscures the view and makes it very easy to accidentally remove the arthroscope from the joint (Fig. 2.45).

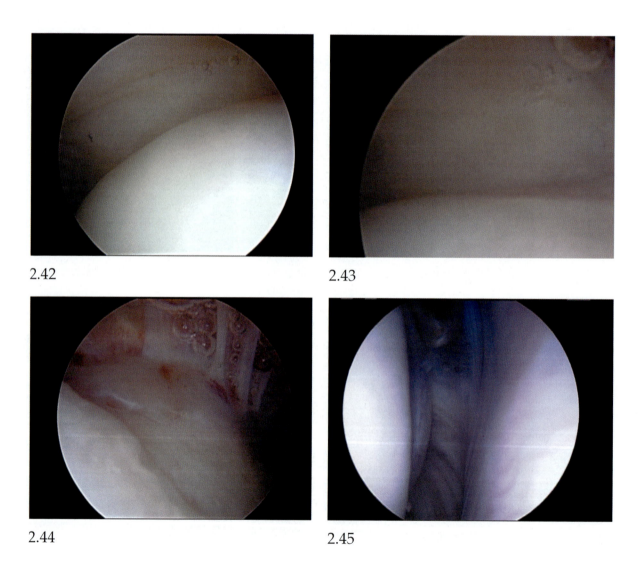

2.42

2.43

2.44

2.45

Inspect the back of the humeral head. Make a gentle rotatory movement of the light source to inspect the whole of the articular surface (Fig. 2.46).

The arthroscope has now come full circle and is back in the starting position. The glenoid and labral examination can now commence. Inspect the anterior labrum and palpate for detachment (Fig. 2.47).

The middle glenohumeral ligament can be seen at this point coming off the anterior anterior labrum and crossing over the subscapularis (Fig. 2.48).

Direct the arthroscope anteroinferiorly to inspect the inferior glenohumeral ligament. At this point it may help to have an assistant place a hand in the axilla to lift the humeral head off the glenoid (Fig. 2.49).

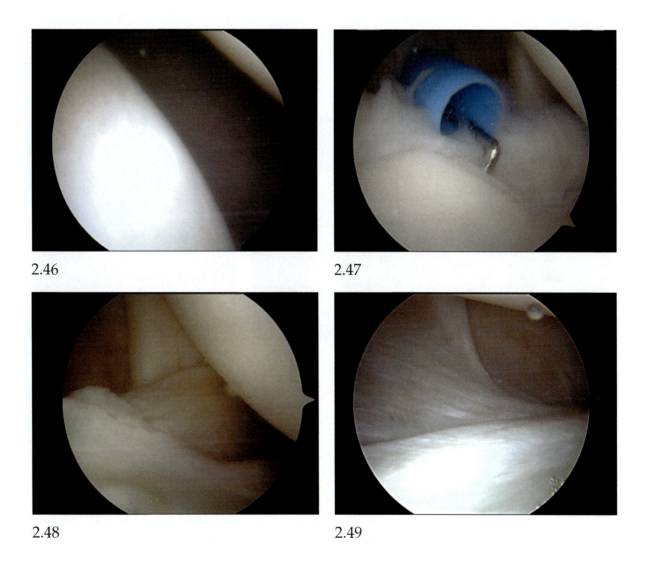

2.46

2.47

2.48

2.49

Inspect the inferior labrum and inferior recess during this manoeuvre (Fig. 2.50).

Withdraw the arthroscope slightly and rotate the light source to see the posteroinferior labrum and posterior glenohumeral ligament (Fig. 2.51).

The posterior labrum up to the biceps anchor can be visualized by carefully withdrawing the arthroscope and rotating the light source (Fig. 2.52).

The basic examination of the glenohumeral joint has now been completed. Re-examine any areas of suspicion. It may be necessary to use the shaver to debride excessive synovial tissue before a firm conclusion can be reached.

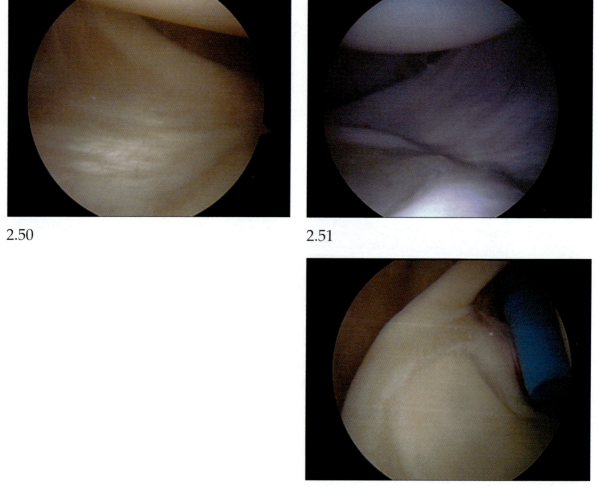

2.50

2.51

2.52

ACROMIOPLASTY

Acromioplasty is one of the most common procedures performed during shoulder arthroscopy and has now all but replaced open acromioplasty as the method of choice for the treatment of subacromial impingement. In our practice we prefer to use the 'cutting block' technique described by Caspari, as this produces consistent results if performed correctly.

The steps to successful acromioplasty start with an appropriately placed lateral portal. This portal must first provide access to the anterior acromion and the coracoacromial ligament, and second must enable a good view of the acromion and the rotator cuff when the instruments are switched and the arthroscope is introduced.

It is worth spending time performing a thorough bursectomy and ensuring that it extends both laterally and posteriorly. When the arthroscope is placed in the lateral portal it becomes very difficult to see the lateral edge of the acromion and the point at which to start the cutting block, if this has not been done.

The key to a smooth and efficient acromioplasty is the development of a smooth cutting block. If this is uneven the irregularities will be propagated as the acromioplasty is developed, particularly if the bone is hard. It is then very difficult and time-consuming to smooth these out later. As the burr approaches the anterior lip of the acromion and the hook try to avoid amputating a large fragment of bone, as this will be difficult to remove. It is far easier to thin the prominence down and then remove it cleanly using the cutting block.

Reinspect the rotator cuff after the acromioplasty has been performed, as it is surprising how often rotator cuff tears become apparent from the lateral portal when they were not visible from the posterior portal.

The patient is positioned on the operating table as described previously. Glenohumeral arthroscopy is performed routinely before the subacromial bursa is approached. It is advisable to create an anterior portal, as this will be beneficial if the rotator cuff is found to be torn.

Introduce the arthroscope into the subacromial bursa. Keep the orientation anatomical, as this will help direct movement. Some surgeons prefer to have the acromion at the top and the rotator cuff inferiorly on the screen, but we feel that this makes orientation more difficult. In this case the acromion is to the left and the cuff to the right (Fig. 2.53).

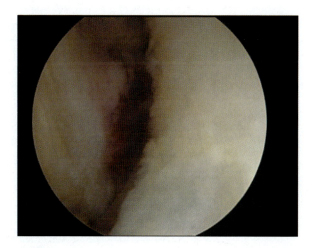

2.53

Make a lateral portal over an 18 g spinal needle as described previously. It is important to confirm that the needle will reach the insertion of the coracoacromial ligament into the acromion (Fig. 2.54).

Using an arthroscopic shaver perform a bursectomy via the lateral portal. It is important to remove bursal tissue posteriorly (towards the arthroscope) and laterally (near the entry point of the shaver) (Fig. 2.55).

Remove soft tissue from the acromion via the lateral portal. This may be performed with the shaver, a burr or a diathermy device. It is advisable to spend some time on this step, as a clear view of the undersurface of the acromion will be required for the acromioplasty step (Fig. 2.56).

Using a diathermy probe, release the coracoacromial ligament and soft tissue from the front of the acromion. If the ligament is detached at the bony insertion there is less risk of bleeding from the coracoacromial artery (Fig. 2.57).

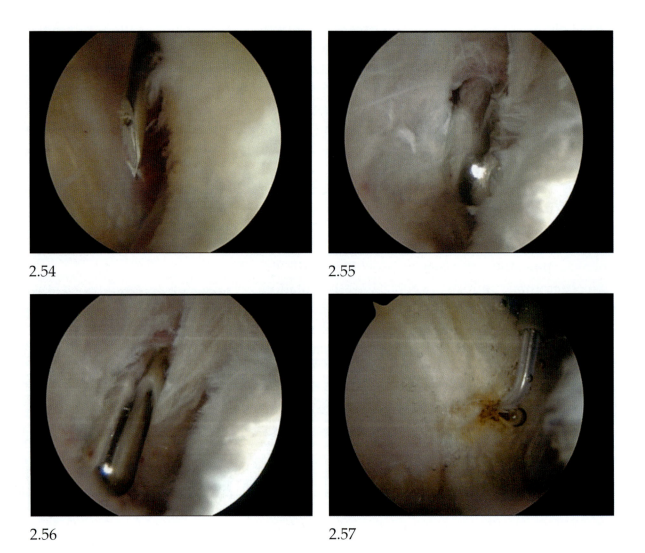

2.54

2.55

2.56

2.57

Remove the thickened periosteum and bursal tissue from the undersurface of the acromion with the shaver or diathermy so that the bone can be seen (Fig. 2.58).

Switch the instruments so that the arthroscope is in the lateral portal. The use of switching sticks makes this step easier. Introduce the burr from the posterior portal. If the undersurface of the acromion has been adequately debrided there should be no need to reintroduce the shaver at this stage (Fig. 2.59).

Lay the burr against the undersurface of the acromion approximately halfway back from the anterior edge and medial, at the junction of the acromioclavicular joint (Fig. 2.60).

If there is residual soft tissue it can be removed with the burr before bone resection is begun (Fig. 2.61).

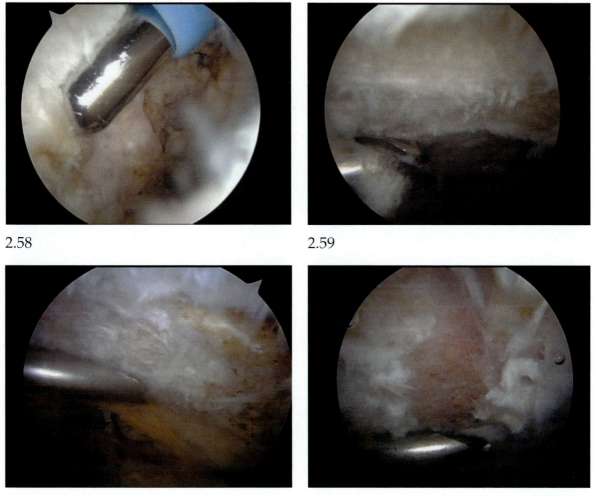

2.58

2.59

2.60

2.61

Use the posterior acromion as a 'cutting block' to guide the amount of resected bone. This is done by laying the shaft of the burr flat against the acromion and allowing it to resect everything proud of that level. For this technique to work the burr must be introduced and laid flat along its length. If the burr is angled up into the acromion, too much anterior bone will be removed (Fig. 2.62).

Advance towards the anterior acromion, sweeping from medial to lateral. Ensure that the resection extends out to the lateral edge of the acromion. If there is residual bursal tissue near the lateral portal this can be difficult to see, but it is important to do so (Fig. 2.63).

If there is a large anterior hook this should be 'thinned' to prevent large fragments separating from the acromion. It is frustrating to remove these fragments once they have separated (Fig. 2.64).

At the completion of the procedure the burr should lie flat on the undersurface of the smooth acromion throughout the length of the resection (Fig. 2.65).

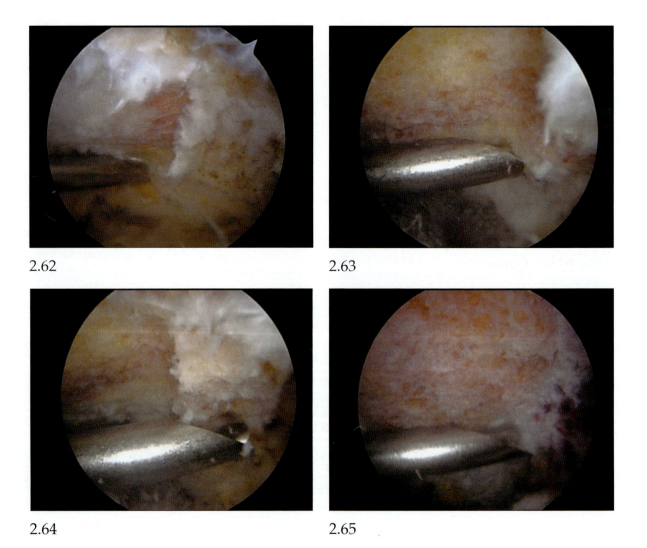

2.62

2.63

2.64

2.65

DISTAL CLAVICLE RESECTION

Distal clavicle excision is usually performed as an adjunct to acromioplasty, although it is possible, and more difficult, to do it without. Time spent early in the procedure performing an adequate bursectomy and removal of the medial fat pad will save time later. Diathermy is usually required, as the fat pad bleeds.

The cutting block technique is used again to excise the distal clavicle, and at the end of the procedure there should be enough room to easily sweep the burr (5.5 mm) in the space created.

The authors recommend that the surgeon be familiar with acromioplasty before attempting distal clavicle resection.

Prepare and position the patient as previously described. Inspect the glenohumeral joint before entering the subacromial bursa. The creation of an anterior portal is recommended while in the glenohumeral joint, as this can be used later if needed.

Reintroduce the arthroscope into the subacromial bursa via the posterior portal and create a lateral portal using a spinal needle as a guide to placement (Fig. 2.66).

Perform a bursectomy and acromioplasty if required. This is described elsewhere in this atlas (Fig. 2.67).

With the arthroscope in the lateral portal and the shaver in the posterior portal debride the bursal tissue and capsule surrounding the inferior aspect of the ACJ. The use of diathermy is often beneficial at this stage, as the fat pad often bleeds considerably. Ensure that the soft tissue resection is continued anteriorly, as the shaver will be reintroduced via this portal (Fig. 2.68).

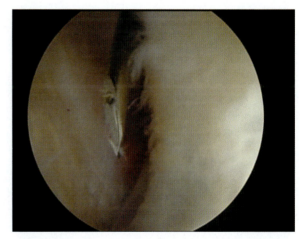

2.66

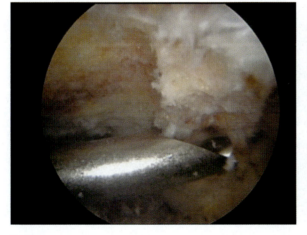

2.67

2.68

Begin the debridement of the visible surface of the ACJ. At this point an assistant applying downward pressure on the distal clavicle improves the view and accessibility. Use a cutting block technique as described for acromioplasty. Try to keep the burr parallel with the surface of the joint and create a cut level off which the rest of the resection can be referenced (Fig. 2.69).

Only a limited resection is possible from the posterior portal. Reintroduce the burr via the anterior portal. It may be easier to remove the blue cannula before this is done. It may also be necessary to reintroduce the shaver and remove more bursal tissue. Continue the excision of the joint using the previously created level as the reference point (Fig. 2.70).

Work from the front of the clavicle to the back, removing slightly more bone than the width of the shaver (Fig. 2.71).

Continue the debridement superiorly until the whole of the clavicle side of the joint has been removed; take care not to breach the superior capsule (Fig. 2.72).

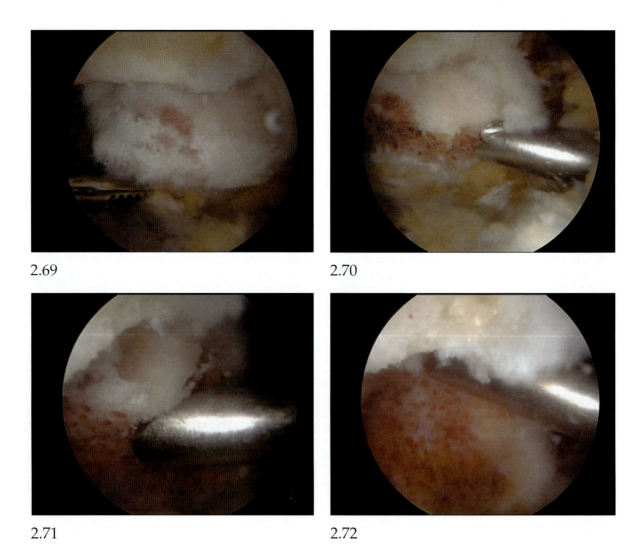

2.69

2.70

2.71

2.72

To improve the view of the superior aspect of the joint, use the burr to remove 1–2 mm of the edge of the acromion. This usually allows the top edge of the clavicle to be seen (Fig. 2.73).

Once finished, it should be possible to visualize the whole of the distal clavicle (Fig. 2.74).

Once the excision has been completed, use the shaver to remove bone debris from the surface of the rotator cuff and reinspect the cuff (Fig. 2.75).

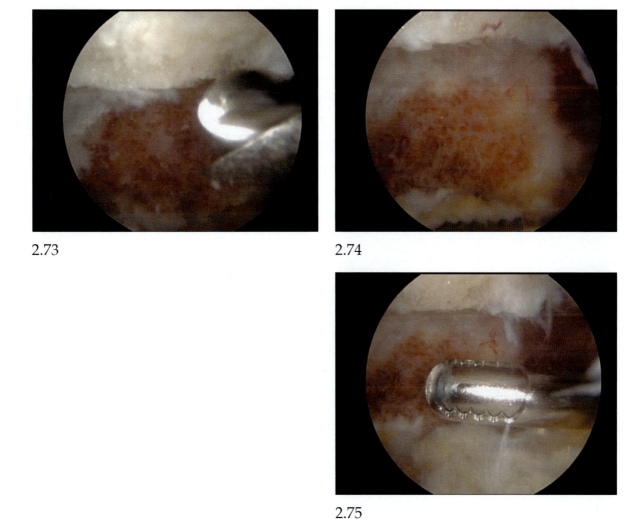

2.73

2.74

2.75

SUPERIOR LABRAL ANTERIOR POSTERIOR (SLAP) REPAIR

The superior labral anterior posterior lesion has only been a truly treatable entity since the advent of arthroscopic surgery. The diagnosis is comparatively easy to make and the treatment principles are simple. As with all arthroscopic procedures involving anchors and sutures the complexity arises with suture management and knot tying. The surgeon must be capable of tying both sliding and non-sliding knots confidently before any anchor work can be undertaken. The anchor type to be used is the personal preference of the surgeon. In our practice we currently use a metal threaded anchor, as it has single step insertion which reduces the chance of slipping and position loss. The anchor comes preloaded with two sutures. Although this has the advantage of reducing the number of anchors that have to be inserted, in many cases the second suture will not slide and a non-sliding knot, such as the Revo, is required.

Other anchors are available, both metal and bioabsorbable. The choice is up to the surgeon.

Prepare and position the patient as previously described. Create a posterior portal and introduce the arthroscope. Create an anterior portal as described and inspect the whole of the glenohumeral joint.

Using a probe, palpate and attempt to lift the biceps anchor off the glenoid. The type II SLAP, in which the biceps anchor and superior labrum have become detached from the glenoid, is amenable to surgical repair (Fig. 2.76).

Replace the probe with a shaver and debride any fibrillated edge of the labrum. This will not only improve the view, but also allows the true labrum to be repaired and sutures to be secure (Fig. 2.77).

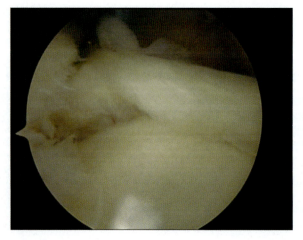

2.76

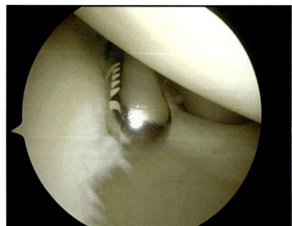

2.77

Use the shaver to remove scar tissue from the undersurface of the biceps anchor. Be careful not to resect any of the biceps insertion. Do not decorticate the glenoid excessively. The 4.5 mm 'aggressive plus' shaver will perform some bone resection, but the burr will often remove more than is desired (Fig. 2.78).

Use an 18 g spinal needle to plan the point of entry of the accessory cannula. The entry point should provide access both anterior and posterior to the biceps anchor (Fig. 2.79).

Make a skin incision and introduce a second cannula into the glenohumeral joint. The cannula will need to be large enough to accommodate a suture anchor (Fig. 2.80).

Concern has been raised about causing damage to the rotator cuff when using this cannula, but little damage appears to occur, as the cannula pierces the muscular portion of the cuff. Alternatively, the anchor can be inserted without a cannula and all the sutures managed through the anterior portal. This can make knot sliding and tying difficult. Another option is to position the cannula in the rotator interval, which makes suture management easier but can make it difficult to work posterior to the biceps.

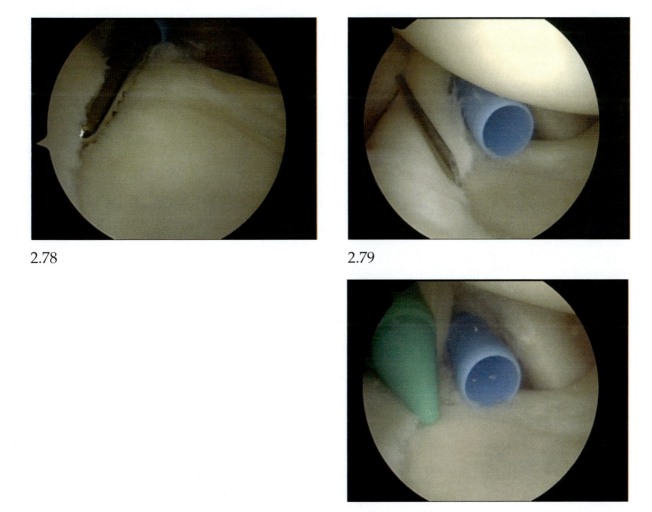

2.78

2.79

2.80

Introduce the suture anchor through the second cannula. Aim to position it at the articular edge of the glenoid. It may be necessary to use a switching stick to move the biceps and labrum posteriorly during this procedure (Fig. 2.81).

We routinely use a 3.5 mm screw-type metal anchor with double sutures. This device has the advantage that it is single-step insertion and no predrilling is required. The double sutures mean that in many cases only a single anchor is required; however, the second suture may not slide after the first has been tied down. Insert the anchor and withdraw the insertion device (Fig. 2.82).

Pass a ring suture grasper through the first (blue) cannula and withdraw all of the sutures (Fig. 2.83).

Pass a 'birdbeak' penetrator through the labrum posterior to the biceps tendon, aiming to exit just superior to the articular surface (Fig. 2.84).

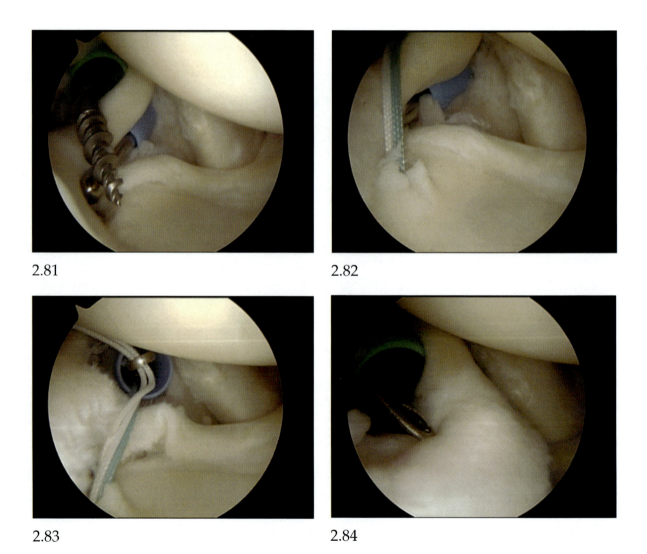

2.81

2.82

2.83

2.84

Grasp a single suture strand. It may help if the assistant uses a grasper to feed the suture into the tissue penetrator's jaws (Fig. 2.85).

Withdraw the suture through the second, superior, cannula (Fig. 2.86).

Using a ring grasper introduced through the second cannula, grasp the free end of the same suture (the one exiting via the anterior cannula) (Fig. 2.87).

Withdraw this through the second cannula. Ensure that the first limb of the suture is not pulled back into the joint as this is done (Fig. 2.88).

Ensure that the suture will glide through the labrum and the anchor. This will determine the type of knot that is used.

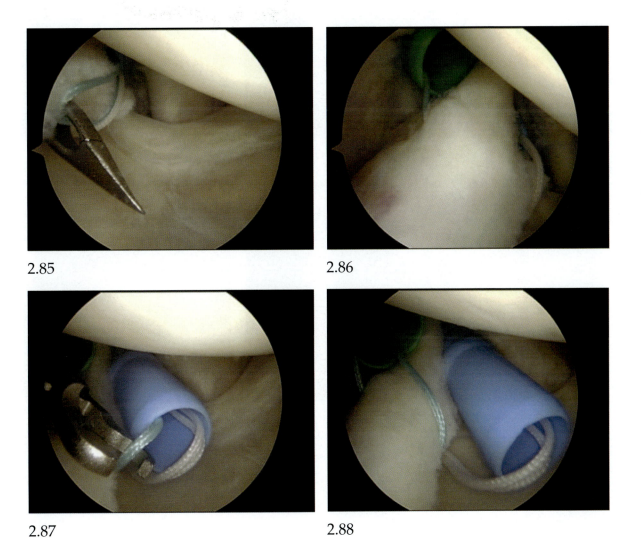

2.85

2.86

2.87

2.88

Tie the suture securely down over the labrum (Fig. 2.89).

Cut the suture ends (Fig. 2.90).

The process is now repeated to secure the anterior portion of the labrum. Pass a 'bird-beak' penetrator through the labrum anterior to the biceps tendon, aiming to exit just superior to the articular surface. Grasp a single suture strand (Fig. 2.91).

Withdraw this suture through the second cannula (Fig. 2.92).

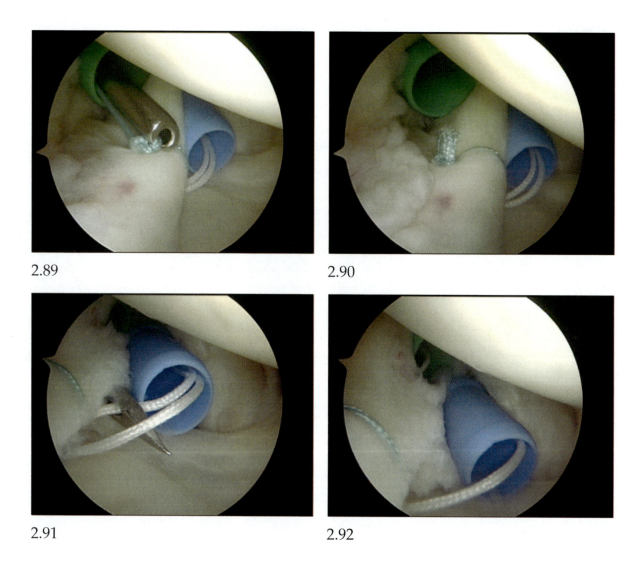

2.89

2.90

2.91

2.92

Grasp the free suture and withdraw this through the second cannula (Fig. 2.93).

Tie the suture down over the labrum (Fig. 2.94).

Cut the suture ends (Fig. 2.95).

At the completion of the procedure the biceps anchor should be securely attached to the glenoid. If there is still instability posteriorly it may be necessary to repeat the procedure with another anchor.

The arthroscope should then be introduced into the subacromial bursa and the examination of the shoulder completed. We tend not to perform acromioplasty at the same time as SLAP repair, as this seems to lead to shoulder stiffness.

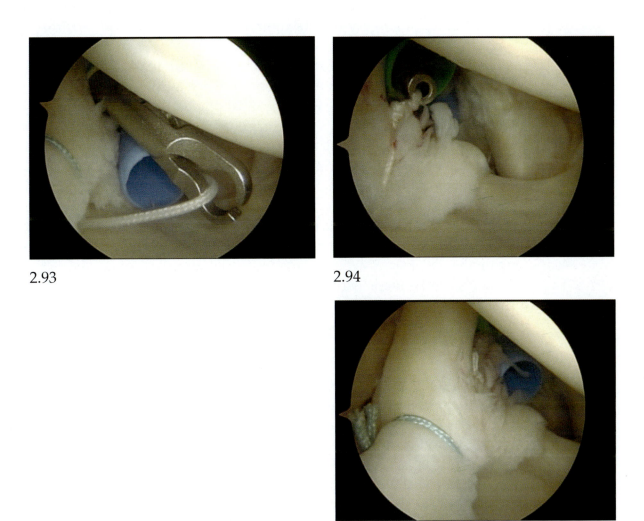

2.93

2.94

2.95

ROTATOR CUFF REPAIR

Tears of the rotator cuff are a common problem which increases with age. Small tears may not be diagnosed prior to surgery, and the arthroscopic surgeon must be prepared to manage them if they are present.

This section describes a number of techniques used during surgery on the rotator cuff. It begins with the technique for passing a suture through the cuff if a partial tear is suspected, enabling both the articular and the bursal surfaces of the same region to be inspected reliably. Margin convergence is a useful technique which, if used appropriately, can make a tear that appears initially to be large into one that may be readily amenable to arthroscopic or open surgery. The technique can be applied both arthroscopically and open.

There are a number of methods for repairing rotator cuff tears arthroscopically. We have described only those that use sutures and bone anchors, as these are not only our preferred techniques but are also those that require the most practice to perform smoothly. There will be other techniques and instruments that can be used. It is important that the arthroscopic surgeon is familiar with a number of alternative techniques to suit differing situations. This means that a variety of equipment must be available for every operation.

The technique of mini-open repair is also described. This has the advantage of being far quicker and technically easier than the arthroscopic technique. Larger tears may not be amenable to entirely arthroscopic techniques, and the mini-open may be more appropriate. It should be borne in mind that if a long time is spent attempting to perform an arthroscopic repair the soft tissue swelling may make an open technique equally challenging. The decision should be made early (usually after debridement of the tear) to save a lot of wasted time.

Suture passing to mark partial-thickness tears

Prepare and drape the shoulder as describe previously. Make standard posterior and anterior portals. Perform a complete glenohumeral joint inspection and treat any other pathology within the glenohumeral joint.

If there is a region of the rotator cuff which is suspicious for a partial-thickness tear use the shaver and gently perform a debridement. This will make the extent of the tear clearer to see (Fig. 2.96).

Using an insertion point just lateral to the edge of the acromion, pass an 18 g spinal needle through the region that is suspicious for a tear. This may take several passes until

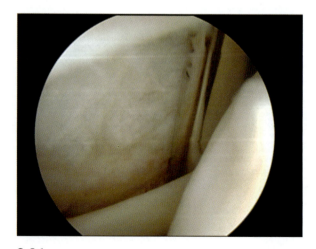

2.96

the correct spot is found. If possible, try to pass the needle perpendicularly through the tear as this will make management of the suture easier in the subacromial space (Fig. 2.97).

Remove the needle from a length of 0 PDS and pass the suture through the needle into the joint (Fig. 2.98).

Grasp the suture and draw it out through the anterior portal. Secure the two ends with a haemostat to prevent it from being inadvertently removed (Fig. 2.99).

Introduce the arthroscope into the subacromial bursa and make a lateral portal over a spinal needle, as described previously. Introduce the shaver and debride bursal tissue so that the cuff can be clearly seen. It is important to debride posteriorly towards the scope and laterally towards the lateral portal. Try to identify the suture as soon as possible, as it is possible to cut through it with the shaver.

Inspect the rotator cuff in the region of the suture. Once this has been done the suture can be removed (Fig. 2.100).

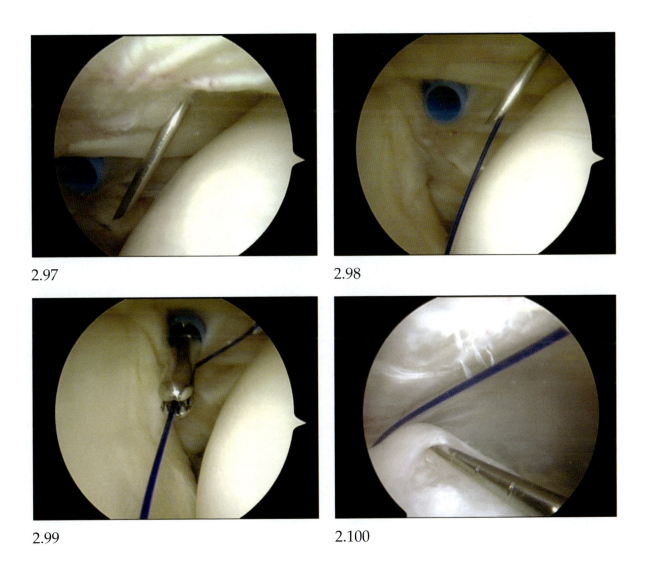

2.97

2.98

2.99

2.100

Mini-open repair

Prepare and drape the patient for shoulder arthroscopy in the lateral decubitus position, as described previously. Introduce the arthroscope using a posterior portal and make an anterior portal using the drive-through technique, also described previously.

Inspect the glenohumeral joint and undertake any procedures that may be required (e.g. SLAP repair) (Fig. 2.101).

Inspect the rotator cuff from the glenohumeral joint side. Here the retracted cuff can be seen on the left of the image. It is often difficult to appreciate the anatomy of a rotator cuff tear from the articular side (Fig. 2.102).

As the rotator cuff can retract and become adherent to the superior glenoid it is important to release it. This can be achieved using a shaver or special rasps, and can be continued through the defect in the cuff once the arthroscope has been introduced into the subacromial bursa (Fig. 2.103).

Introduce the arthroscope into the subacromial bursa and create a lateral portal as described. Perform a bursectomy. Do not spend a long time on this as it can be continued using scissors if the procedure is converted to mini-open, and the soft tissues will become engorged making the procedure more difficult.

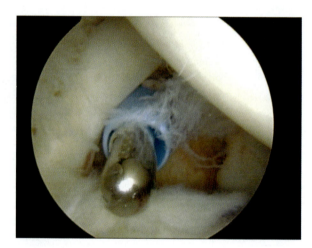

2.101

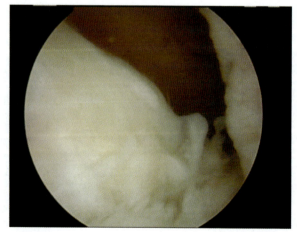

2.102

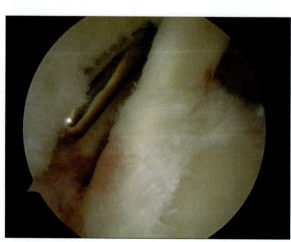

2.103

At this stage the cuff tear can be assessed and the decision made whether to proceed with an arthroscopic or a mini-open repair (Fig. 2.104).

Perform a subacromial decompression as described previously. This is an essential part of the rotator cuff repair and will improve visualization. Again this must be done quickly, as the longer the arthroscope is in the bursa the more soft tissue distension will result (Fig. 2.105).

Remove the instruments from the bursa and express excess fluid.

The skin incision for a mini-open repair is approximately 4 cm long and is centred on the incision made previously for the lateral arthroscopy portal. The incision extends proximally as far as the lateral edge of the acromion. It is important not to detach the deltoid from the acromion. The incision is continued through the subcutaneous fat, and the deltoid muscle is split (Fig. 2.106).

These images are orientated so that the arm and greater tuberosity are superior and the free edge of the rotator cuff is inferior.

Insert a shoulder surgery retractor. Here a Charnley-type retractor is being used (Fig. 2.107).

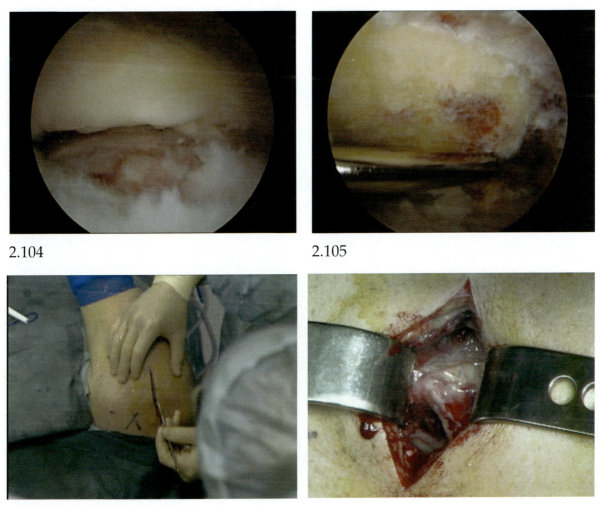

2.104

2.105

2.106

2.107

There will still be a significant amount of bursal tissue and this should be removed with scissors (Fig. 2.108).

Further mobilization of the cuff is performed either with a finger or using a blunt periosteal elevator. The release should be extended proximally in the anterior, superior and posterior portions of the cuff (Fig. 2.109).

A single traction suture may be helpful in determining the mobility of the cuff and the correct position of the reduction. Define the edges of the cuff tear and assess the morphology. In this case the tear is predominantly crescent shaped; however, there is a small almost longitudinal extension posteriorly (Fig. 2.110).

Plan the repair before inserting the suture anchors. In this case the posterior portion of the tear will be repaired using margin convergence sutures (side–side), and two 5 mm metal screw-type suture anchors will be inserted for the reattachment of the cuff.

Use a burr to debride the greater tuberosity, but do not decorticate excessively (Fig. 2.111).

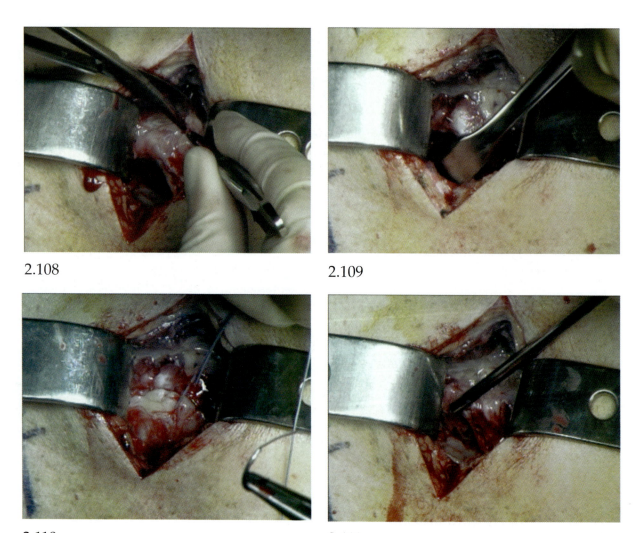

2.108

2.109

2.110

2.111

The margin convergence is undertaken first as this will reduce the tension when the repair to bone is undertaken. Using the traction suture to maintain the correct position place a single simple suture through the two free edges of the rotator cuff (Fig. 2.112).

Place a second suture if necessary. In this case it is anterior to the first and has been left untied to allow access to the greater tuberosity for the rest of the procedure (Fig. 2.113).

Reassess the extent of the cuff detachment and determine the suture anchor requirement and position (Fig. 2.114).

We routinely use a 5 mm double-suture screw-type metal anchor because it requires only single-step insertion and provides two sutures for every anchor inserted. In this example the anchor has been inserted into the posterior aspect of the exposed greater tuberosity (Fig. 2.115).

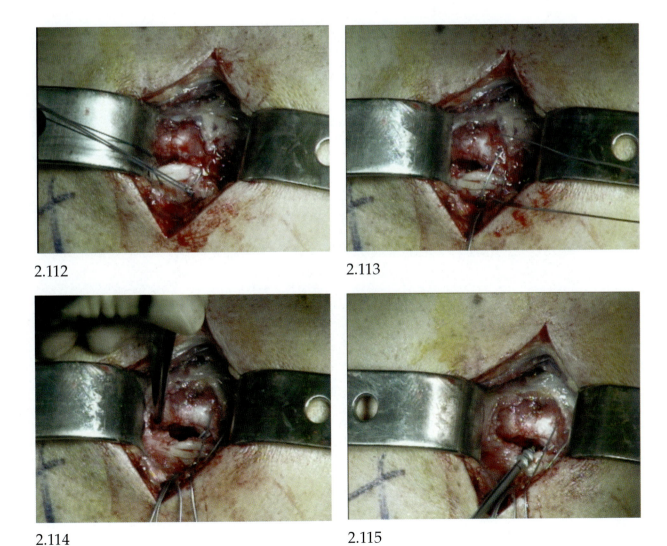

2.112

2.113

2.114

2.115

Arrange the sutures to facilitate management. The green sutures will be passed second and they are laid down the arm to keep them free of the white sutures. The first white suture to be passed is threaded on to a Mayo needle; the second is laid down the arm but separate from the green sutures (Fig. 2.116).

Pass the first limb of the white suture through the free edge of the cuff to exit on the superior surface (Fig. 2.117).

Pass the second limb in a similar fashion to form a mattress suture. The two limbs are not tied at this time (Fig. 2.118).

Pass the first limb of the green suture in the same manner (Fig. 2.119).

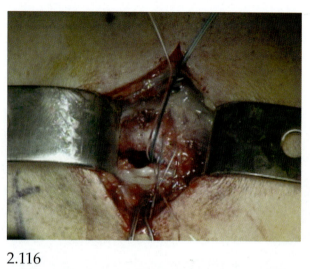

2.116

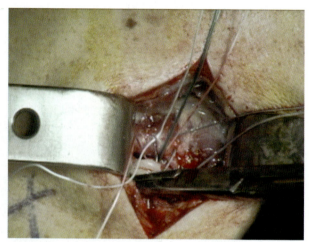

2.117

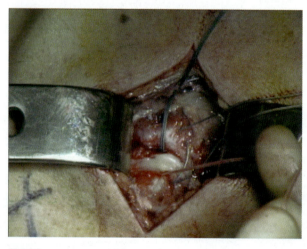

2.118

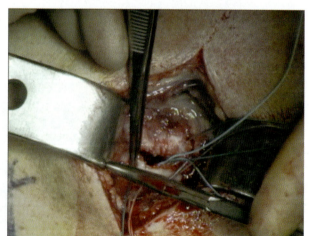

2.119

Pass the second limb of the green suture to form a second mattress suture. Again this is not tied at this time (Fig. 2.120).

If a second anchor is required, insert it at this stage. In this case a second anchor has been inserted anterior to the first anchor (Fig. 2.121).

Remove the insertor to expose the sutures (Fig. 2.122).

Arrange the sutures in the same way as before, with the green sutures running down the arm (Fig. 2.123).

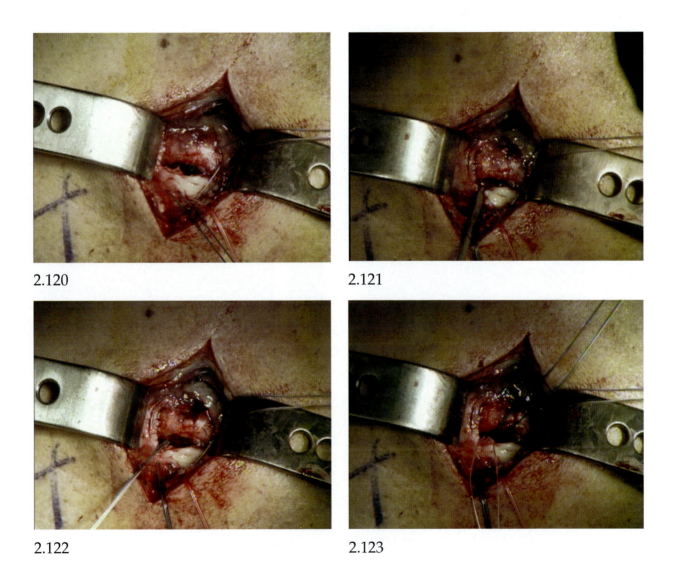

2.120

2.121

2.122

2.123

Pass the white sutures in a mattress fashion but do not tie them at this stage (Fig. 2.124).

Pass the green sutures in the same manner. There is now one posterior margin convergence suture which has been tied and a second which has not. There are four mattress sutures securing the cuff to the greater tuberosity, and these also have not been tied (Fig. 2.125).

Now tie the five sutures securely reattaching the rotator cuff to the greater tuberosity with little or no tension (Fig. 2.126).

Irrigate the wound and close the deltoid fascia with 2/0 Vicryl. Close the skin in layers as preferred (Fig. 2.127).

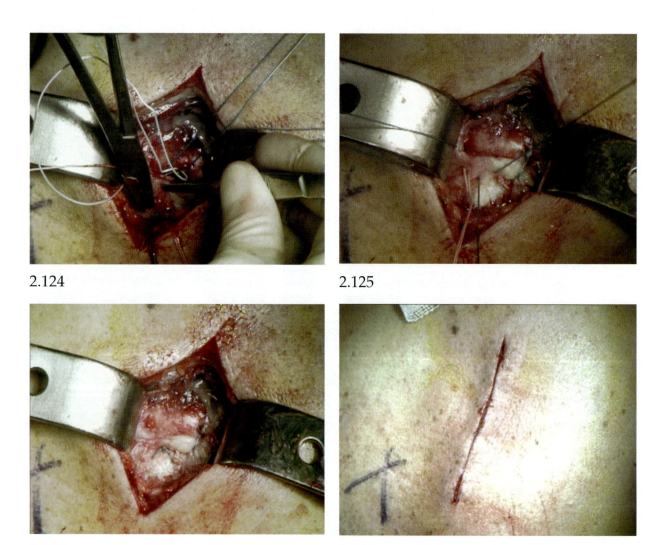

2.124

2.125

2.126

2.127

Margin convergence

The patient is placed on the operating table in the lateral decubitus position and prepared for standard shoulder arthroscopy. Create a posterior and an anterior portal using a drive-through technique. Inspect the whole of the glenohumeral joint and treat any pathology.

Reintroduce the arthroscope into the subacromial bursa and create a lateral portal over a spinal needle, as described previously. Perform a bursectomy and acromioplasty if necessary.

Inspect the region of the rotator cuff tear. If the tear has a linear component, i.e. it is L-shaped instead of a simple C-shaped tear, it may be amenable to margin convergence before the repair to bone (Fig. 2.128).

Take time to inspect and understand the morphology. Inspection from the lateral portal can help. If this step is rushed it can make the subsequent repair difficult and the chance of failure greater.

If you have not already done so, introduce the arthroscope through the lateral portal.

Load a birdbeak suture passer with no. 2 Ethibond and introduce it from the posterior portal (Fig. 2.129).

Pass the birdbeak through the posterior leaf of the rotator cuff. Ensure that the bite is adequate and the suture will not pull out later (Fig. 2.130).

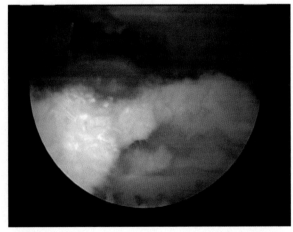

2.128

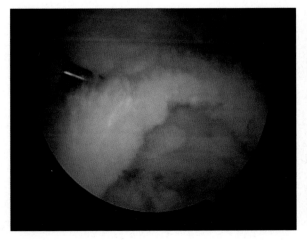

2.129

2.130

Angle the birdbeak and pass it through the anterior leaf until the grasper is clear (Fig. 2.131).

Introduce a ring grasper from the anterior portal and pass off the Ethibond from the suture passer to the ring grasper (Fig. 2.132).

Release the suture from the birdbeak and withdraw it before any movement is made with the grasper (Fig. 2.133).

The suture should pass under the cuff tear, as illustrated (Fig. 2.134).

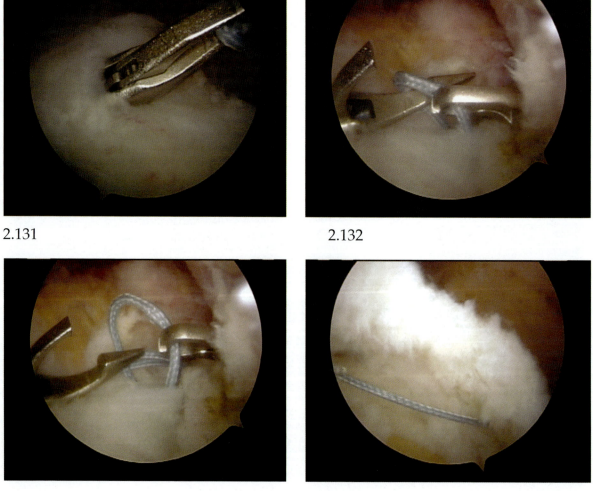

2.131

2.132

2.133

2.134

The suture limbs can then be tied down (Fig. 2.135).

This process can be repeated until the longitudinal limb of the tear has been closed. The tear can then be repaired to the greater tuberosity, as described in the relevant section (Fig. 2.136).

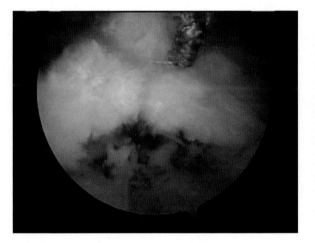

2.135

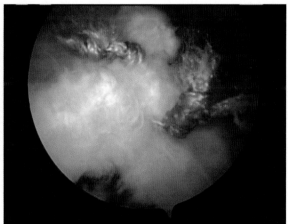

2.136

ARTHROSCOPIC ROTATOR CUFF REPAIR

Prepare and drape the shoulder as described previously. Make posterior and anterior portals and inspect the glenohumeral joint. Undertake any treatment within the joint at this time. If there is a region of the articular side of the rotator cuff which is suspicious for a partial-thickness or a complete tear, pass a suture as described elsewhere.

Introduce the arthroscope into the subacromial bursa and make a lateral portal over a spinal needle, as described.

Perform a bursectomy and subacromial decompression as described. This will improve visualization of the tear and allow access for repair (Fig. 2.137).

Start with the arthroscope in the lateral portal. This gives the best overall view of the tear and allows for better appreciation of the tear anatomy. It may be necessary to move the arthroscope between the portals as the procedure progresses to allow better visualization and easier working (Fig. 2.138).

Switch the arthroscope to the posterior portal. This step may be facilitated by the use of switching sticks. Debride the edges of the cuff tear using a shaver (Fig. 2.139).

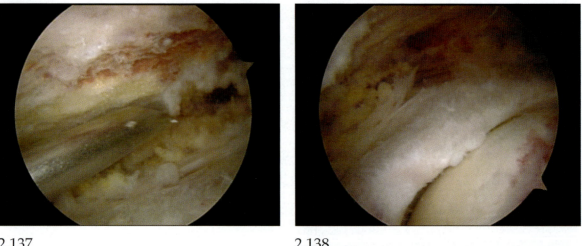

2.137

2.138

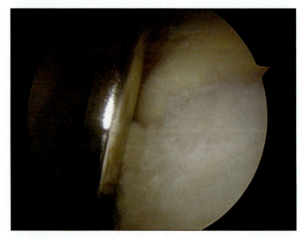

2.139

Cuff mobility must be assessed to determine whether it can be repaired directly to the greater tuberosity or if further mobilization is needed. This may be done with a grasper (Fig. 2.140).

Alternatively, pass a Caspari suture punch loaded with 0 PDS from the lateral portal and grasp the lateral edge of the cuff (Fig. 2.141).

Withdraw the punch, leaving the suture through the cuff. The cuff mobility can now be tested. This technique has the advantage that if the suture is left in place traction can be applied to the cuff as needed (Fig. 2.142).

Introduce a burr through the lateral portal and decorticate the greater tuberosity. This should not be excessive, as the bone quality is often poor (Fig. 2.143).

Determine the best access for the suture anchor. The anchor should be directed medially at the 'deadman's angle'. It may be possible to use the existing lateral portal by enlarging it. It may be necessary to make an additional portal close to the lateral one: an accessory portal.

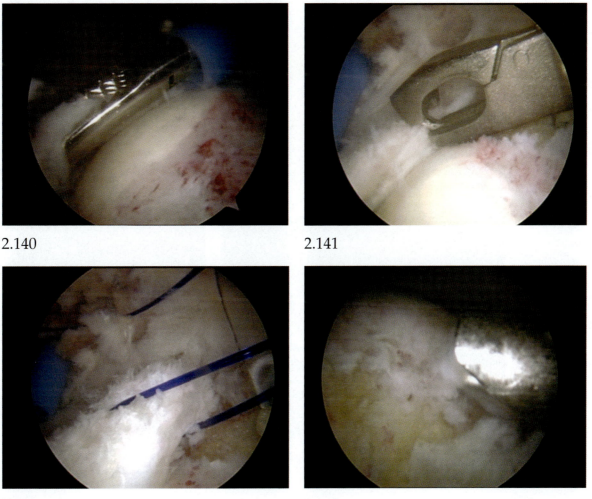

2.140

2.141

2.142

2.143

We prefer to use a 5 mm metal screw-type anchor with double sutures. This device has the advantage that it is single-step insertion and no predrilling is required. The double sutures mean that in many cases only a single anchor is required; however, the second suture may not slide after the first has been tied down. Insert the anchor and withdraw the insertion device, in this case via the lateral portal (Fig. 2.144).

Withdraw the sutures through the portal. Confirm the security of the anchor before the procedure is continued, as poor bone quality may result in anchor pullout (Fig. 2.145).

Withdraw one of the white sutures via the accessory portal (Fig. 2.146).

The next step is to pass one limb of the white suture through the cuff. If a PDS suture is in place the undersurface limb can be tied to the PDS and pulled through the cuff. In this picture from another case the two limbs of the Caspari suture can be seen entering the cannula with a single limb of the white suture (Fig. 2.147).

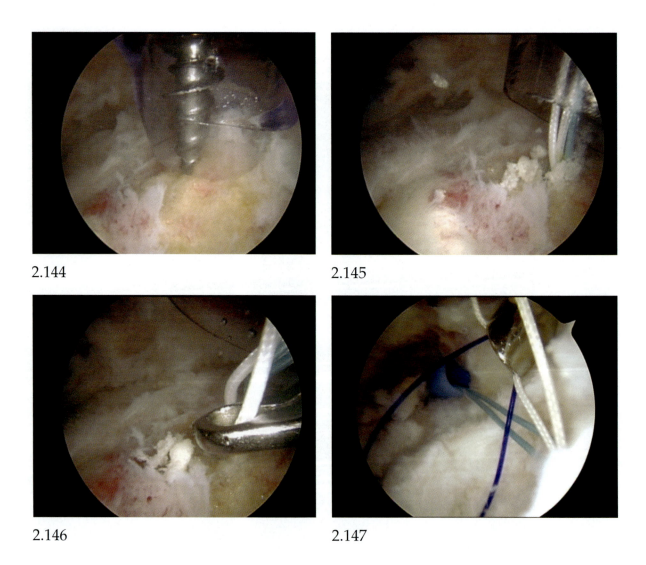

2.144

2.145

2.146

2.147

Tie the PDS and the white suture together. Draw the white suture through the cuff by the Caspari suture (Fig. 2.148).

An alternative technique is to load the suture on to a birdbeak tissue penetrator and pass it through the cuff from the inferior to the superior surface (Fig. 2.149).

If this is done it may be necessary to use a ring grasper to take the limb out of the jaws of the tissue penetrator and through the anterior portal (Fig. 2.150).

For suture management and tying, bring this limb back so that it exits via the accessory portal (Fig. 2.151).

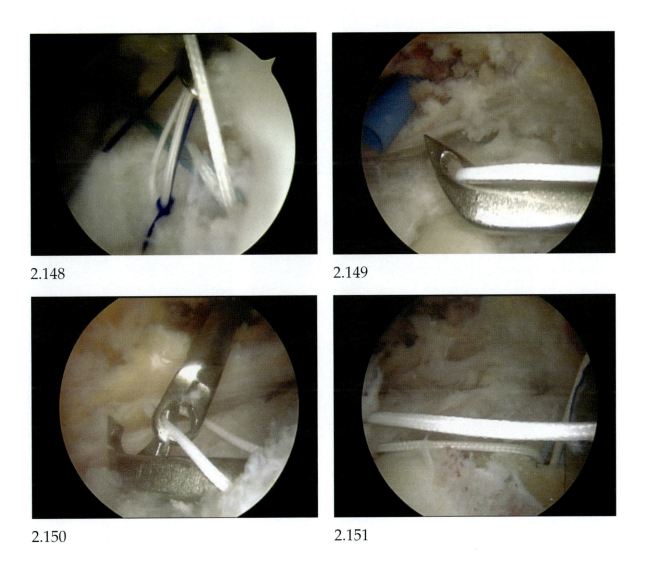

2.148

2.149

2.150

2.151

If both limbs are not through the accessory portal, use the ring grasper to bring them together (Fig. 2.152).

The cuff can now be pulled over the humeral head using the white suture (Fig. 2.153).

This suture can now be tied; however, it is advisable to pass the second suture before tying, as it becomes very difficult to pass an instrument through the cuff if a secure repair has been done with one limb. In this case the white sutures are being taken out through the lateral portal (Fig. 2.154).

This allows the green sutures to be grasped from the accessory portal (Fig. 2.155).

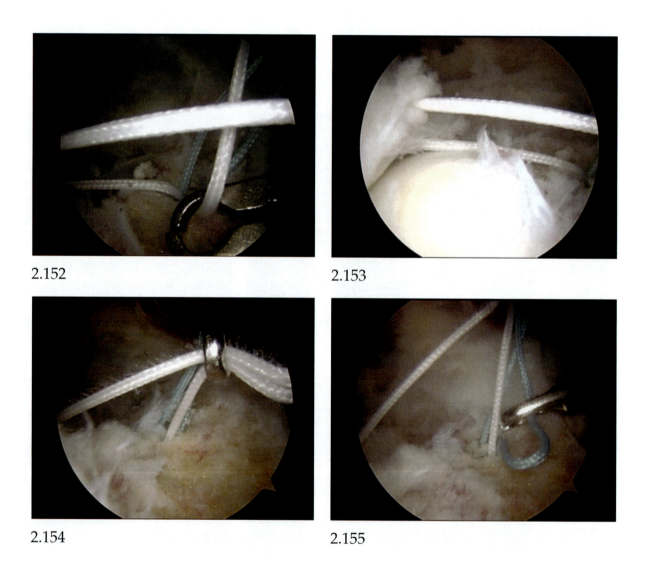

2.152

2.153

2.154

2.155

The white sutures exit through the lateral portal and the green through the accessory portal. This keeps the sutures from becoming tangled (Fig. 2.156).

For this suture a Caspari suture punch has been used to pass the suture through the cuff, although any of the suture passing techniques can be used (Fig. 2.157).

The white suture is still through the lateral portal; the green sutures exit through the accessory portal, as do both limbs of the Caspari suture (Fig. 2.158).

The first (white) suture can now be tied without compromising the passage of the second suture, and making suture management easier (Fig. 2.159).

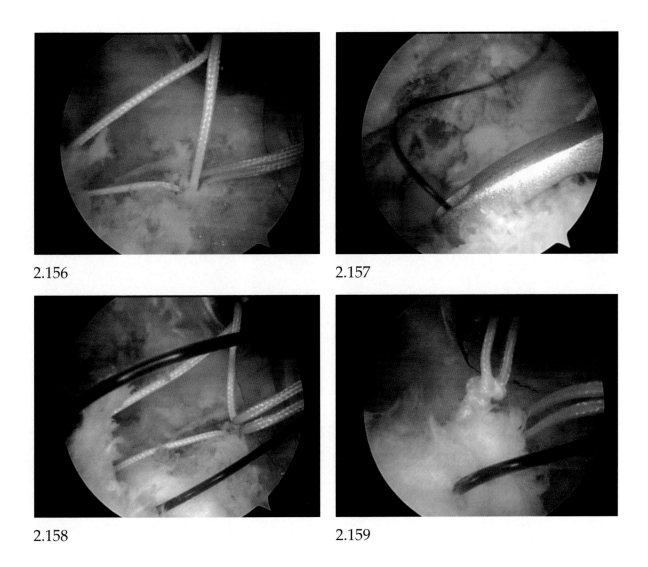

2.156

2.157

2.158

2.159

Tie the undersurface limb of the Caspari suture to one limb of the green suture and pull it through the cuff. Before this is done it is advisable to pass the ring grasper down one suture limb to ensure that they are not twisted (Fig. 2.160).

Tie the green suture over the cuff (Fig. 2.161).

If the cuff repair is felt to be inadequate a second suture anchor may be inserted if desired. This is done in the same manner as the first (Fig. 2.162).

The same process is followed until the cuff repair is secure, although it may not be necessary to use both limbs of a double-loaded anchor (Fig. 2.163).

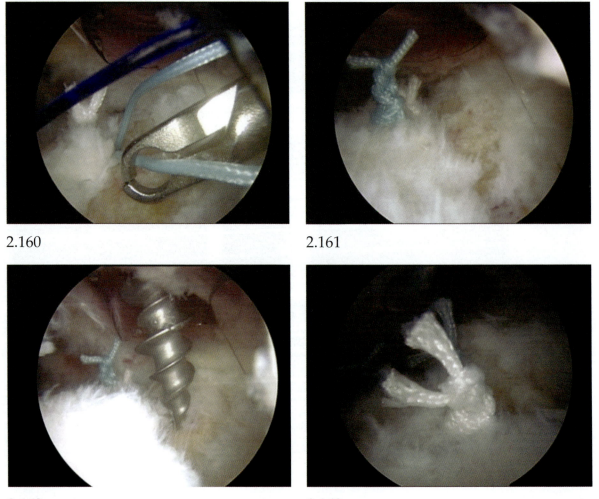

2.160

2.161

2.162

2.163

INSTABILITY SURGERY

Shoulder instability is a relatively frequent problem in the younger population. The gold standard of surgery has traditionally been open techniques. Arthroscopic techniques are equally effective but they must be performed correctly.

This section describes the techniques of Bankart repair and capsular shift. The technique of transglenoid repair (originally described by Caspari) is also described. It is useful to be familiar with this technique because, if the anchors fail during a standard Bankart repair, transglenoid sutures may enable the repair to be completed successfully.

It is important to position the patient as described in the relevant section to enable good access to the joint during surgery. The relevant anatomy and potential for neurological damage must be appreciated to avoid damage during portal placement.

Rotator interval closure

Prepare and drape the shoulder as described previously. Make posterior and anterior portals and inspect the joint. Perform any other procedures that may need to be undertaken within the glenohumeral joint.

Introduce a long 18 g spinal needle into the joint just anterior to the biceps tendon. This may pierce the anterior edge of the supraspinatus tendon (Fig. 2.164).

Pass a length of no. 0 PDS through the needle into the joint (Fig. 2.165).

Direct the blue cannula in the anterior portal so that it lies behind the free edge of the subscapularis tendon (Fig. 2.166).

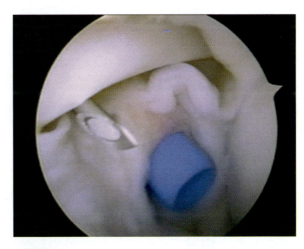

2.164

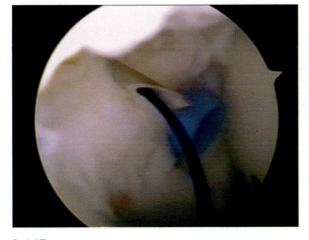

2.165

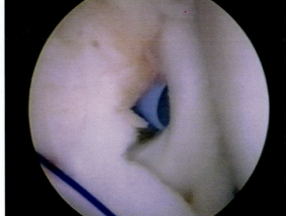

2.166

Pass a suture capturing device such as a birdbeak tissue penetrator through the anterior cannula so that the free edge of the subscapularis is pierced (Fig. 2.167).

Grasp the PDS suture with the tissue penetrator. It is often helpful to direct the suture with the spinal needle into the jaws of the penetrator. Withdraw the suture through the sub-scapularis tendon and secure the two ends with a haemostat (Fig. 2.168).

If a second suture is required this can be passed using the same technique. Insert a long 18 g spinal needle in a position to complement the first, and again pass a length of no. 0 PDS suture through the needle (Fig. 2.169).

Withdraw the suture through the anterior cannula using the tissue penetrator (Fig. 2.170).

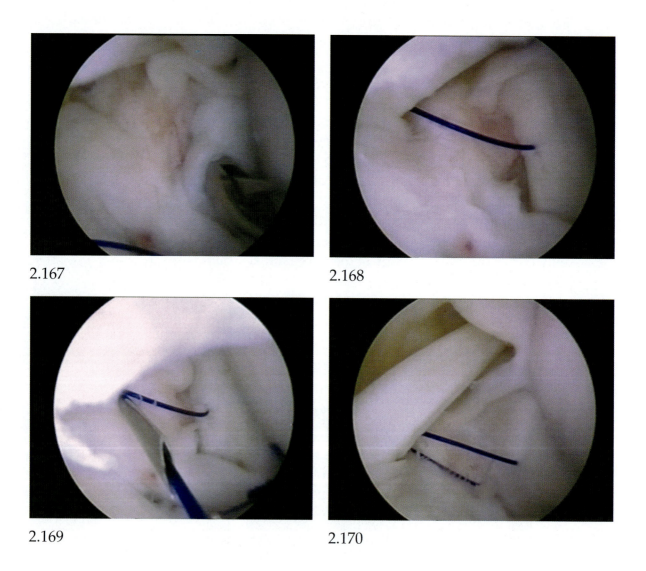

2.167

2.168

2.169

2.170

When the sutures are pulled tight the rotator interval is closed (Fig. 2.171).

An alternative technique is to pass a long spinal needle down the anterior cannula to pierce the free edge of subscapularis (Fig. 2.172).

Pass a length of PDS suture into the joint (Fig. 2.173).

Withdraw the cannula slightly and redirect it so that a birdbeak suture passer can be passed through the anterior edge of supraspinatus (Fig. 2.174).

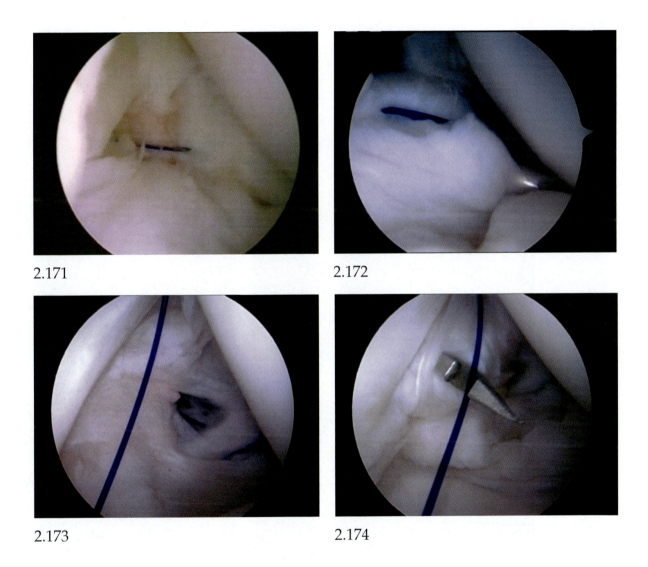

2.171

2.172

2.173

2.174

Grasp the suture using the tissue penetrator, withdrawing it so that it spans the rotator interval (Fig. 2.175).

As the suture is drawn tight the rotator interval is closed (Fig. 2.176).

An alternative method of tying the suture which ensures that the deltoid muscle is not caught up in it is to tie it under direct vision in the subacromial bursa.

The arthroscope is introduced into the subacromial bursa and a lateral portal is created over a spinal needle, as described previously. The blue cannula is then identified anteriorly. If the cannula is kept firmly in the capsular tissue a shaver can be used to debride bursal tissue without risk of cutting the sutures (Fig. 2.177).

Tie the sutures within the cannula (Fig. 2.178).

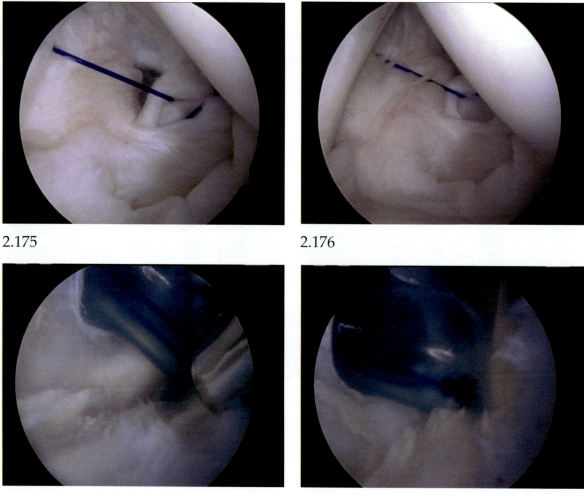

2.175

2.176

2.177

2.178

Cut the sutures, leaving them securely tied over the capsule and rotator interval tissue but not over the deltoid (Fig. 2.179).

Capsular shift

Prepare and drape the patient as described previously. Create a posterior and an anterior portal in the described fashion.

Inspect the whole of the glenohumeral joint. For capsular shift to be an appropriate operation there should be no evidence of a Bankart lesion (i.e. an intact labrum). Capsular laxity with a drive-through sign should be seen. The anteroinferior capsule will be lax and the IGHL may be absent (Fig. 2.180).

If it has not already been done, create an anterior portal.

Using a shaver, release the capsule from the glenoid. This should be started approximately 5 mm from the neck. Continue the release through the capsule until subscapularis is seen (Fig. 2.181).

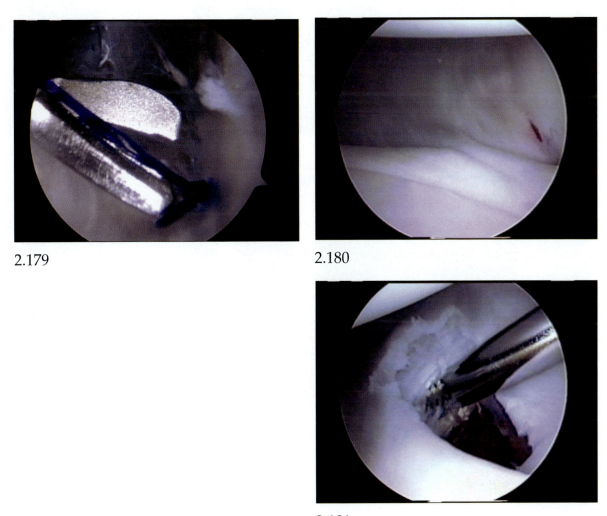

2.179

2.180

2.181

The inferior aspect of the release should extend down to the 6 o'clock position.

The proximal limit of the release should be the level of the free border of subscapularis (Fig. 2.182).

Exchange the cannula for one large enough to accommodate a Caspari suture punch. A 7.5 mm cannula will allow the use of an open or 'Snyder'-type Caspari punch (Fig. 2.183).

Load the suture punch with 0 PDS and pass it through the inferior capsule at the 6 o'clock position (Fig. 2.184).

Withdraw the punch. The open type will leave one limb of the suture in the joint (Fig. 2.185).

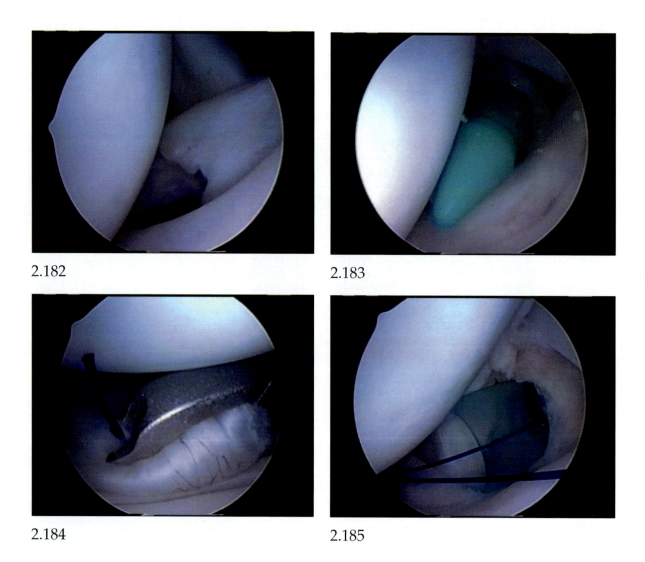

2.182

2.183

2.184

2.185

Pass a birdbeak-type tissue penetrator through the free edge of subscapularis, grasp the free limb of the suture and withdraw it (Fig. 2.186).

To facilitate suture management it is often easier to reposition the cannula so that the first suture limbs are outside it. This reduces the risk of tangling the sutures when the second is passed. The sutures must be reinserted before any knots can be tied (Fig. 2.187).

Pass a second 0 PDS suture through the inferior capsule using the Caspari suture punch (Fig. 2.188).

Retrieve the free end using a birdbeak suture passer through the subscapularis, as before (Fig. 2.189).

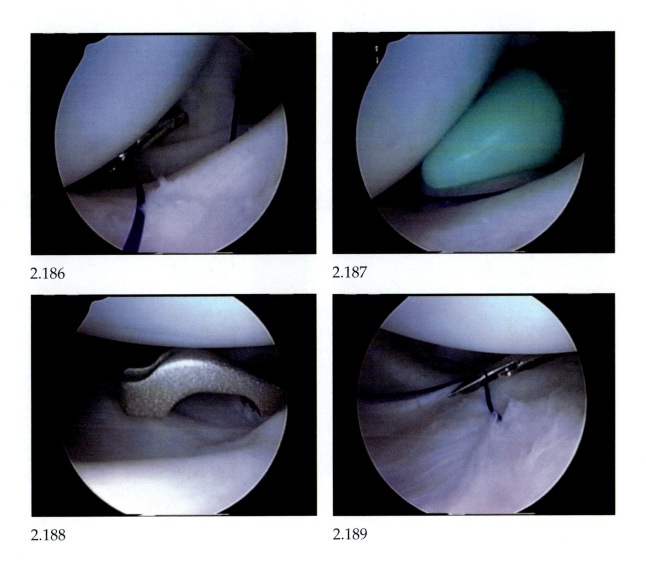

2.186

2.187

2.188

2.189

Reposition the cannula so that all four limbs are inside. It is important that the cannula always passes through the original site. If a second track is created a soft tissue bridge will be formed, preventing the knots from being tied (Fig. 2.190).

Tie down both of the sutures on to subscapularis. This will draw the inferior capsule up towards the free border (Fig. 2.191).

Close the rotator interval as described previously, using one or two sutures (Fig. 2.192).

Once the rotator cuff has been closed it should appear as here (Fig. 2.193).

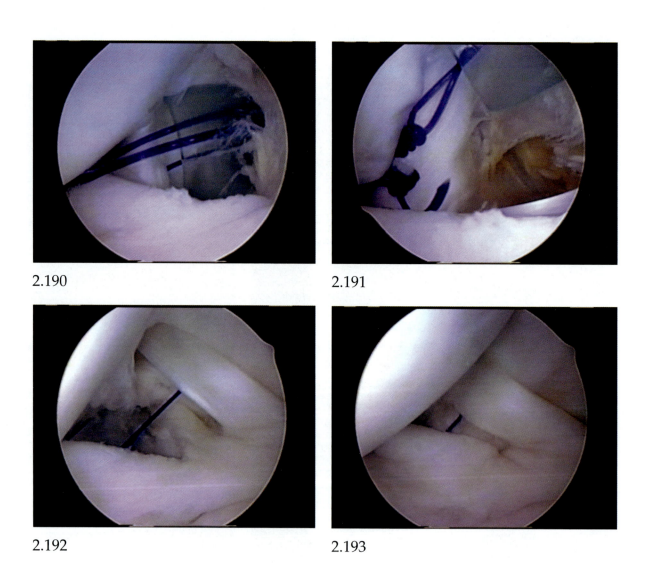

2.190

2.191

2.192

2.193

The drive-through sign will then be obliterated and the anteroinferior capsular redundancy will be taken up (Fig. 2.194).

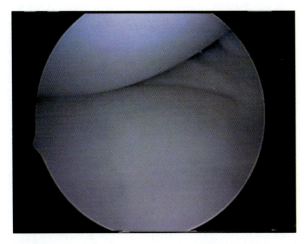

2.194

ANTERIOR STABILIZATION

Bankart repair – bone anchor technique

Prepare and drape the patient as for routine shoulder arthroscopy. Create a posterior portal and introduce the arthroscope. Create an anterior portal as described, using the drive-through technique.

Inspect the whole of the glenohumeral joint. If instability is suspected pay careful attention to the anterior labrum and capsule. The Bankart lesion often reattaches to the glenoid neck, therefore it is important to pay careful attention to the position of the labrum. In this case the tear is fresh and the detachment can be clearly seen (Fig. 2.195).

Two anterior portals will be required. Use a spinal needle to identify the correct position for the accessory anterior portal. It is essential that this portal allows access to the inferior aspect of the labrum (Fig. 2.196).

Detach the labrum from the glenoid neck. This can be done using a shaver, a banana blade or a number of specially designed instruments, such as the elevator shown (Fig. 2.197).

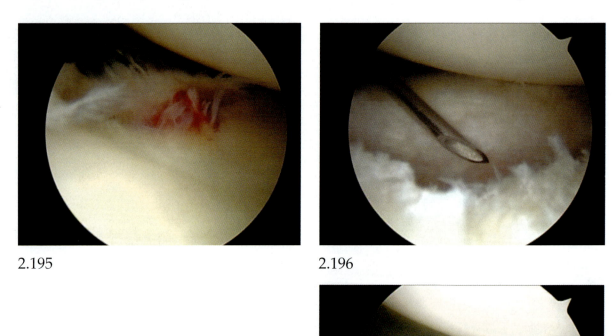

2.195

2.196

2.197

The detachment must be continued round past the 6 o'clock position to allow the inferior capsule to be pulled up (Fig. 2.198).

The release must be continued down until subscapularis is seen. Only in this way can the capsule be shifted sufficiently to reattach it to the edge of the glenoid. It is apparent when an adequate release has been performed, as the anterior labrum/capsule falls away from the glenoid (Fig. 2.199).

Once the soft tissues have been detached from the glenoid use a burr or shaver to prepare the bone. Extensive decortication is not required, but a raw surface is necessary to promote reattachment (Fig. 2.200).

Plan the position of the suture anchors using a probe or switching stick. Aim to place the inferior anchor as close to the 6 o'clock position as possible, and to keep the anchors as perpendicular to the face of the glenoid as possible (Fig. 2.201).

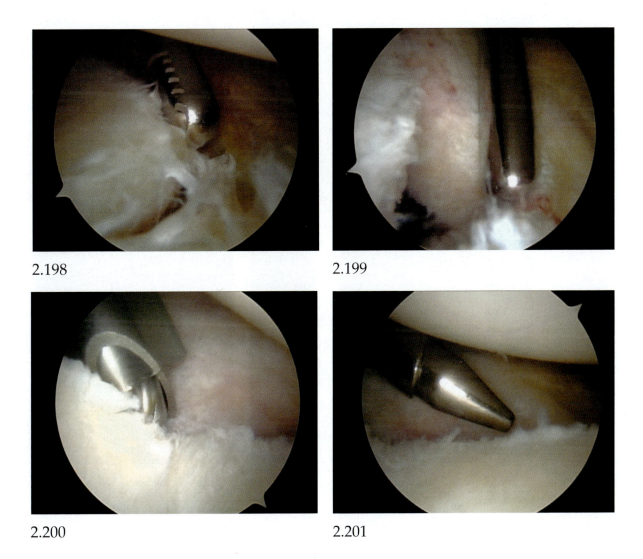

2.198

2.199

2.200

2.201

Use a suture-passing device to insert a suture in the capsule at the 6 o'clock position. This allows traction to be put on the capsule and will be used to pull through the suture attached to the suture anchor (Fig. 2.202).

This step is far easier to perform before any suture anchors have been placed, and facilitates the correct placement of the anchor in relation to the position of the suture in the capsule (Fig. 2.203).

The first anchor can now be positioned and inserted. In this case a prethreaded bioabsorbable has been used, which requires predrilling (Fig. 2.204).

The anchor can then be driven home. Note the position, which is just on the articular surface of the glenoid. Do not try to reattach the labrum to the glenoid neck, as this will not provide sufficient stability later (Fig. 2.205).

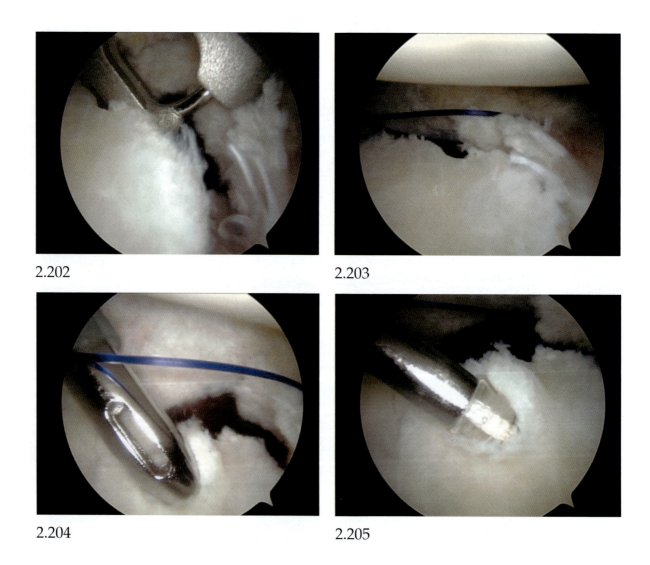

2.202

2.203

2.204

2.205

Remove the introducer, leaving the two suture tails of the anchor. A ring passer can then be used to isolate and withdraw one of the limbs (Fig. 2.206).

Tie this limb to the inferior limb of the previously passed traction suture and use the latter to pull the anchor suture through the labrum. Tie the suture down over the labrum. Note the buttress effect created by the positioning of the anchor on the face of the glenoid rather than the neck (Fig. 2.207).

Repeat the process to place a second anchor. First the traction suture is passed through the labrum in the 4–5 o'clock position (Fig. 2.208).

Insert the second anchor in the corresponding position on the glenoid. Note that this is slightly higher than the position of the traction suture, so that the labrum will continue to be drawn up the glenoid neck. In this illustration the anchor has been inserted and the introducer is being withdrawn (Fig. 2.209).

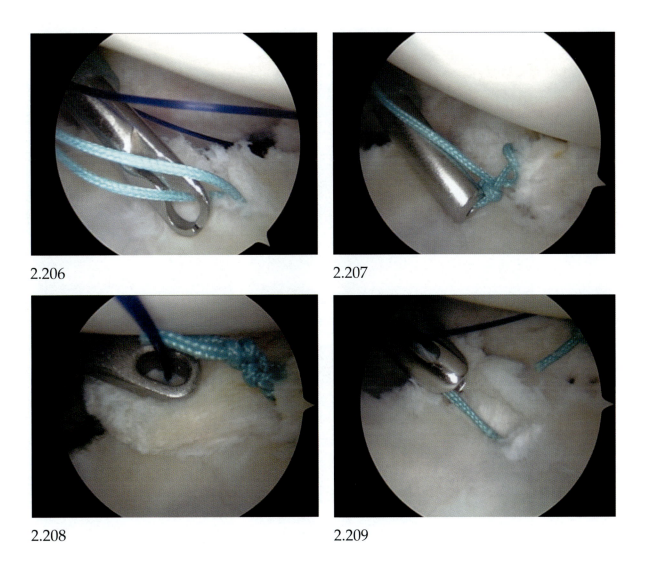

2.206

2.207

2.208

2.209

As described previously, use the traction suture to pull one limb of the anchor suture through the labrum (Fig. 2.210).

Tie down the second suture. Again, note the buttress effect created (Fig. 2.211).

Repeat the process with a third suture anchor in the 3 o'clock position (Fig. 2.212).

At this level no traction can be placed on the labrum and it is therefore not necessary to place a traction suture. A tissue penetrator can therefore be used to retrieve one of the suture limbs (Fig. 2.213).

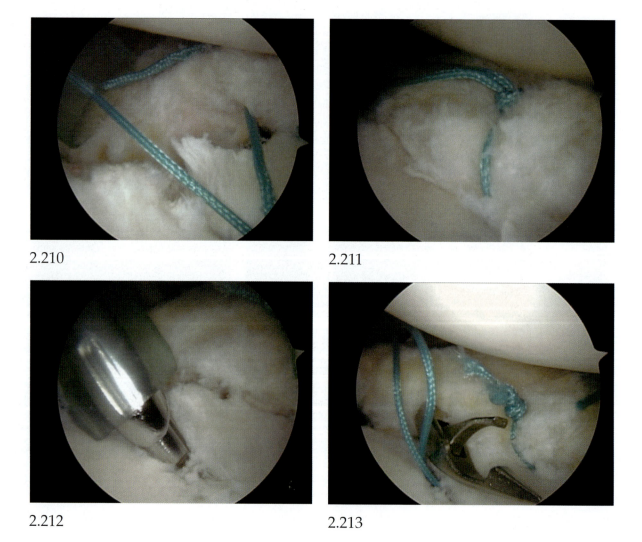

2.210

2.211

2.212

2.213

Tie down the third suture (Fig. 2.214).

At this point the repair is complete. Note the buttress effect of the repair and the position of the anchors in the 3–6 o'clock positions (Fig. 2.215).

Bankart repair – transglenoid technique

The patient is prepared and draped as for standard shoulder arthroscopy. It is important for this technique to ensure that the glenoid face is parallel to the floor for ease of orientation. The posterior drape must also be low enough to allow access to the scapular spine. At least one assistant is required, but two is easier.

Create a posterior portal as described previously and introduce the arthroscope. Make a full inspection of the joint and create an anterior portal using the drive-through technique, as described. The position of the portal in relation to the free edge of the subscapularis tendon is not critical using this technique.

The Bankart lesion is often partially reattached to the glenoid neck and must be released before it can be attached in the correct position. This can be done using a banana blade (Fig. 2.216).

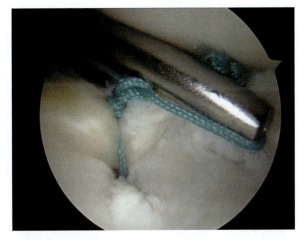

2.214

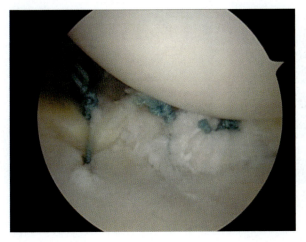

2.215

2.216

Keeping the edge of the blade against the glenoid neck, develop the release down to beyond the 6 o'clock position (Fig. 2.217).

Then use a shaver to develop the release down the neck. Debride the scar tissue but do not extensively decorticate the glenoid neck (Fig. 2.218).

The release must be continued until subscapularis muscle is seen. If this is not done it will not be possible to pull the capsule proximally (Fig. 2.219).

Introduce the slotted transglenoid cannula via the anterior portal. The advantage of this cannula is that it will allow a Caspari suture punch to pass through it while the jaws are still open. At this stage it is helpful to have an assistant lift the humeral head away from the glenoid by placing a hand in the axilla (Fig. 2.220).

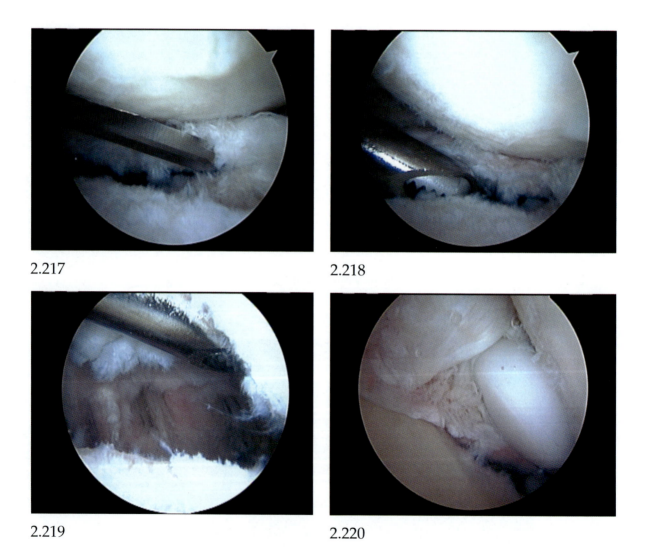

2.217

2.218

2.219

2.220

Load a Caspari suture punch with no. 0 or 2 PDS and insert it through the cannula. Working sequentially from anterior to inferior allows for easier suture management. Grasp the detached labrum with the suture punch and work the needle through the tissue (Fig. 2.221).

Feed the suture through the needle until 1 cm remains outside the suture punch (Fig. 2.222).

Open the jaws of the punch and free the needle from the tissue. Withdraw the punch, taking care to take both ends of the suture with it. The slotted cannula is designed for this step. If it is not used the cannula will have to be removed with the punch and reinserted for the next suture. Once outside the body, secure the suture ends with a haemostat (Fig. 2.223).

Repeat the procedure until sutures have been placed down to the 6 o'clock position. Secure all the sutures together with a haemostat (Fig. 2.224).

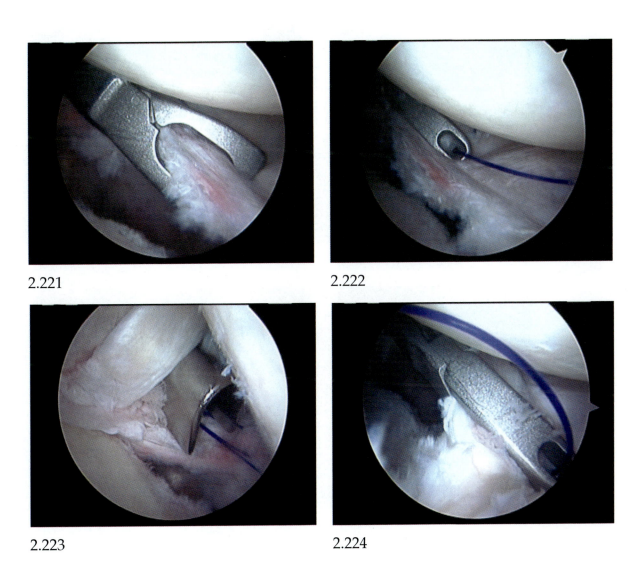

2.221

2.222

2.223

2.224

Once all of the sutures have been placed (usually six or more) the whole of the labrum will move as one if the sutures are tensioned (Fig. 2.225).

Introduce the transglenoid drill guide and position it so that one of the two holes is adjacent to the glenoid, just off the face (Fig. 2.226).

The transglenoid drill is a 4.5 mm drill with a tip slightly wider than the shaft. The proximal end has an eye for suture passage. Aim the drill so that the exit point is below the scapular spine and medial to the glenoid neck. This avoids damage to the suprascapular nerve as it runs over the posterior glenoid neck (Fig. 2.227).

Advance the drill until it tents the skin and incise over the tip. Dissect down with finger and haemostat until the fascia overlying the infraspinatus is identified (Fig. 2.228).

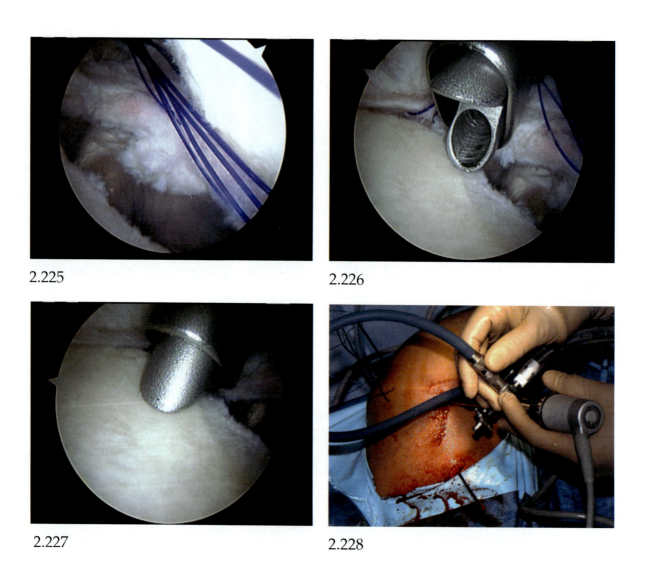

2.225

2.226

2.227

2.228

Pass a length of no. 5 Ethibond through the eye of the drill bit and tie it in a loop. Position the knot so that it is close to the eye. Pass the PDS sutures through the Ethibond loop (Fig. 2.229).

Pull the drill bit through the scapula, drawing the transglenoid sutures with it using the Ethibond loop (Fig. 2.230).

Once the sutures are through, complete any blunt dissection to free the fascia around them (Fig. 2.231).

Divide the sutures into two bundles. There is no need to separate them into corresponding limbs. Thread one bundle on to a free needle and make a single pass through the fascia, entering as close to the exit point as possible. When this is repeated with the other bundle a fascial bridge is created between the two bundles (Fig. 2.232).

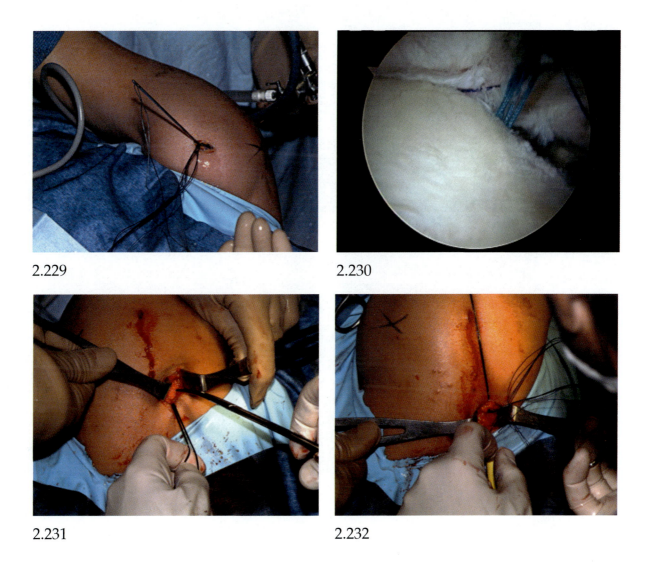

2.229

2.230

2.231

2.232

Tension each of the suture limbs individually; this ensures that all lengths start at the same approximate tension. It is helpful to give the tensioned limbs to an assistant (Fig. 2.233).

Internally rotate the humerus: this will take the tension off the anterior capsule, allowing the sutures to be finally tensioned firmly. The capsule and labrum will be seen to ride up proximally over the glenoid face. This is normal (Fig. 2.234).

Take one length from each bundle and tie them together firmly over the rest of the sutures. This will lock the sutures in place without creating a bulky mass (Fig. 2.235).

Once the knot has been tied, cut the excess suture and close the skin in layers (Fig. 2.236).

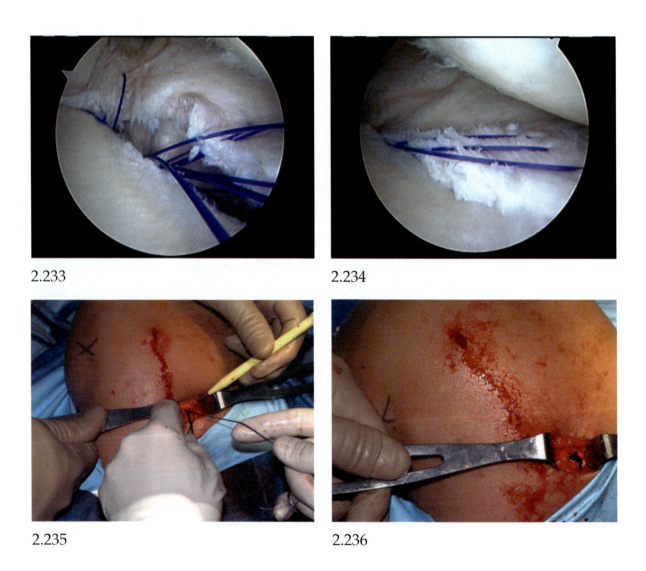

2.233

2.234

2.235

2.236

The completed stabilization is not routinely inspected as this can create undue tension, as it is difficult to see without externally rotating the humeral head. In this example the arthroscope has been reintroduced via the anterior portal. Several of the sutures can be seen overlying the glenoid face. This is normal and does not result in any long-term problems (Fig. 2.237).

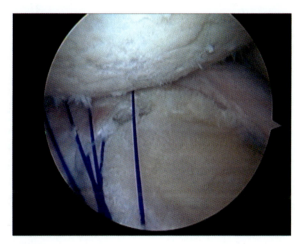

2.237

3 ELBOW ARTHROSCOPY

INTRODUCTION

Arthroscopy of the elbow is performed far less frequently than on the shoulder or the knee. There are pitfalls associated with the technique, as neurovascular structures are in close proximity to the elbow. Knowledge of the anatomy is essential, as is careful portal placement and creation. Once the portals have been created switching sticks should be used to ensure that they are maintained. If the portals are lost once the soft tissues have started to distend they are very difficult to recreate.

Access to the joint is limited and a knowledge of the intra-articular anatomy is required.

Only patient setup, portal creation and the normal arthroscopic examination are described in this chapter. Simple procedures such as loose body removal do not need to be described here, and more complex procedures are performed infrequently. They are not described and are outside the scope of this atlas.

As with the rest of this book the preferred techniques of the authors are described. It is possible to arthroscope the elbow in both the lateral and the prone positions, and both have advantages in certain circumstances. We feel that the supine position we have described is the easiest to set up and use, but we would encourage surgeons to try the alternatives and decide which works best in their hands.

Neurovascular risks

The anterolateral portal lies very close to the radial nerve as it courses close to the radial head. The posterior branch of the lateral cutaneous nerve of the forearm (LCNF) is also at risk. The LCNF arises as the terminal branch of the musculocutaneous nerve and divides into an anterior and a posterior branch. The posterior branch runs over the lateral epicondyle of the humerus and is therefore at risk.

The anteromedial portal lies between the medial cutaneous nerve of the forearm and the median nerve and brachial artery. As the trocar pierces pronator teres and flexor digitorum profundus the median nerve is 1 cm lateral, with the brachial artery in close proximity. As the trocar progresses deeper it is 6 mm from the median nerve in the undistended elbow and 10 mm in the distended elbow; 90° of flexion are also essential to maximize this distance. The ulnar nerve lies behind the medial epicondyle and care must be taken not to damage this, particularly when using instruments via a posterior portal.

The posterolateral portal carries similar risks to the anterolateral portal in relation to the lateral cutaneous nerve of the forearm and the posterior cutaneous nerve, but the radial nerve is at little risk in this approach.

PATIENT SETUP

Elbow arthroscopy is routinely performed under general anaesthesia. This may be supplemented by an axillary block. The patient is placed supine on the operating table and positioned with the operation-side shoulder at the edge of the table. A tourniquet is applied, but if the arm is too short and the tourniquet may impede surgery it should be removed before the case starts (Fig. 3.1).

Exsanguinate the arm using an Eschmark bandage (Fig. 3.2).

Prepare the arm with iodine from the wrist to the tourniquet (Fig. 3.3).

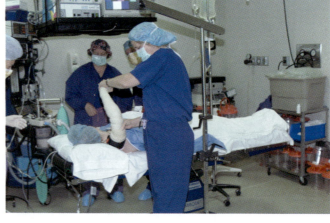

3.2

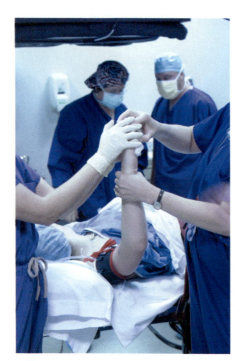

3.1

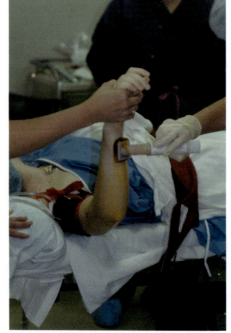

3.3

Place a U-drape under the arm and bring the tails together round over the tourniquet (Fig. 3.4).

Place a sterile stockinette over the hand in the same manner as for shoulder arthroscopy. If there is excess material this should be cut off, as it will interfere with surgery (Fig. 3.5)

Secure the stockinette with a sterile bandage, which should stop approximately 5 inches distal to the elbow (Fig. 3.6).

Complete draping using an extremity drape with a rubber dam (Fig. 3.7).

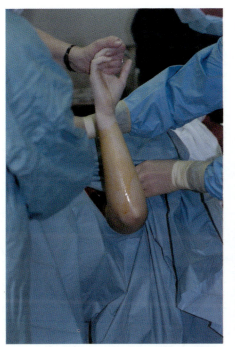

3.4

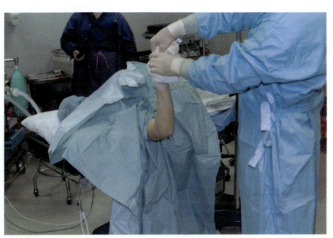

3.5

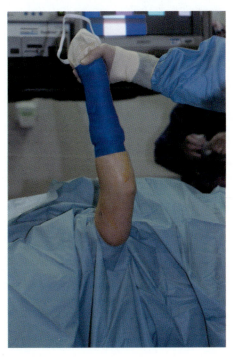

3.6

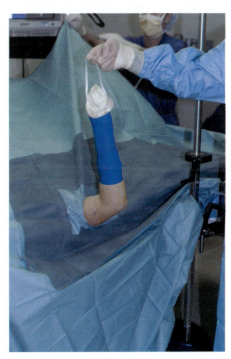

3.7

Traction can then be applied to the elbow: 5 lb is usually sufficient. The traction apparatus used is the same as that for the shoulder. A gentle tug down at the elbow after the weights have been attached will improve the traction (Fig. 3.8).

To complete the sterile area wrap a shutoff drape round the traction upright and the pulley cord (Fig. 3.9).

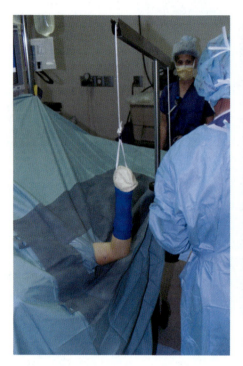 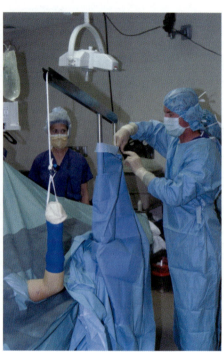

3.8   3.9

PORTAL PLACEMENT

Because of the close proximity to the elbow of a number of neurovascular structures it is essential to mark the anatomical landmarks prior to any portal placement. Also, it is easy to become disorientated when learning elbow arthroscopy, and the skin markings provide a reference (Fig. 3.10).

On the radial side, mark the radial head and the lateral epicondyle (Fig. 3.11).

On the medial side, mark the position of the ulnar nerve and the medial epicondyle. Palpate the tip of the olecranon, but it is not essential to mark this structure (Fig. 3.12).

A reliable and safe entry point into the joint is the soft spot located proximal and inferior to the radial head, between this and the lateral border of the olecranon. Insert a 16 g needle through this spot and inject 10–15 ml saline into the joint. Position can be confirmed by disconnecting the syringe. If the injection is into the joint backflow will be seen (Fig. 3.13).

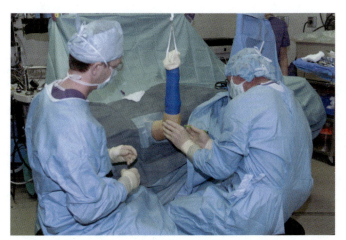

3.10

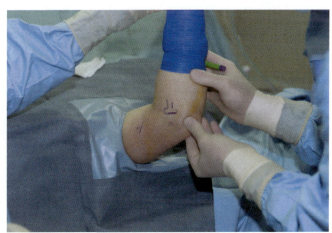

3.11

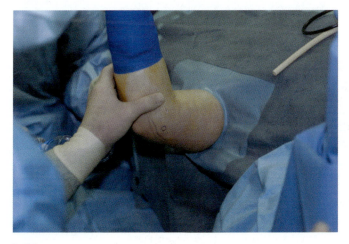

3.12

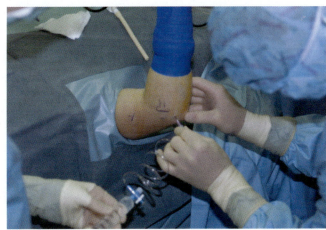

3.13

Once the joint has been distended the portals can be created. Some surgeons prefer to create a lateral portal over the radial head. However, the authors feel that it is easy to create this portal too close to the radial head, which makes access difficult, and we therefore create the medial portal first and the lateral portal second. The medial portal is located 2 cm proximal and 2 cm anterior to the medial epicondyle. Make a skin incision only by drawing the skin over the tip of a no. 11 blade and blunt dissect down to the capsule (Fig. 3.14).

A standard 4.5 mm arthroscope is used, as this provides a larger field of view. Introduce a blunt trocar down to the level of the capsule. Direct the trocar laterally, across the face of the humerus, and push it through the capsule. If bone can be felt with the trocar tip the neurovascular structures will be safe and no damage will be caused to the anterior aspect of the humerus. If the sleeve is within the joint, removing the trocar will result in backflow of saline (Fig. 3.15).

Introduce the arthroscope. Our preference is for a 4.5 mm 30º arthroscope, as we are most familiar with this and it gives a large field of view (Fig. 3.16).

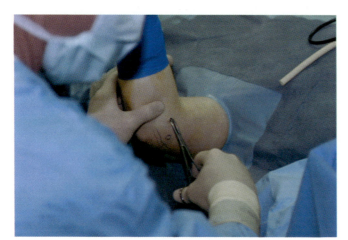

3.14

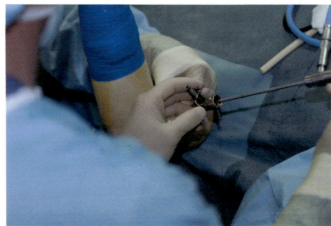

3.15

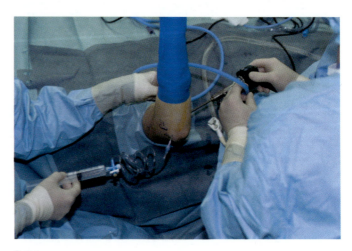

3.16

Create the lateral portal using a spinal needle to confirm placement. The landmark is 2 cm anterior and 3 cm distal to the lateral epicondyle. If the needle enters the joint directly at the level of the radial head the radial nerve will be safe. This technique also allows confirmation that any instruments will be able to reach all appropriate areas of the joint (Fig. 3.17).

Using the same skin incision and blunt dissection technique, create the lateral portal (Fig. 3.18).

Insert a short 4.5 mm blue cannula through the lateral portal. If this is removed at any stage during the operation it will be very difficult to recreate the same portal in the same place (Fig. 3.19).

Instruments can then be introduced via the lateral portal (Fig. 3.20).

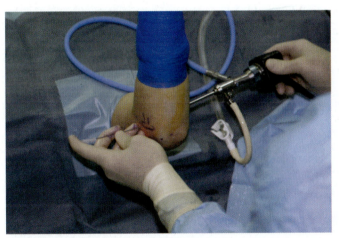

3.17

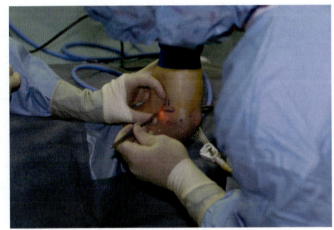

3.18

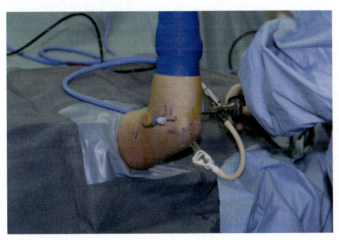

3.19

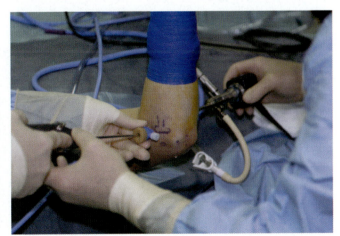

3.20

If you wish to switch portals and introduce the arthroscope via the lateral portal, the simplest technique is to use a switching stick introduced via the lateral portal. This can be done with or without the cannula in situ (Fig. 3.21).

Release the arthroscope from the sleeve and withdraw it slowly, following the switching stick as you direct it up the arthroscope sleeve (Fig. 3.22).

The arthroscope sleeve can then be removed, as the switching stick now runs in through the lateral portal, across the joint and out through the medial portal (Fig. 3.23).

Slide the arthroscope sleeve over the lateral end of the switching stick and the plastic cannula over the medial end before the arthroscope and any instruments (in this case a shaver) are introduced (Fig. 3.24).

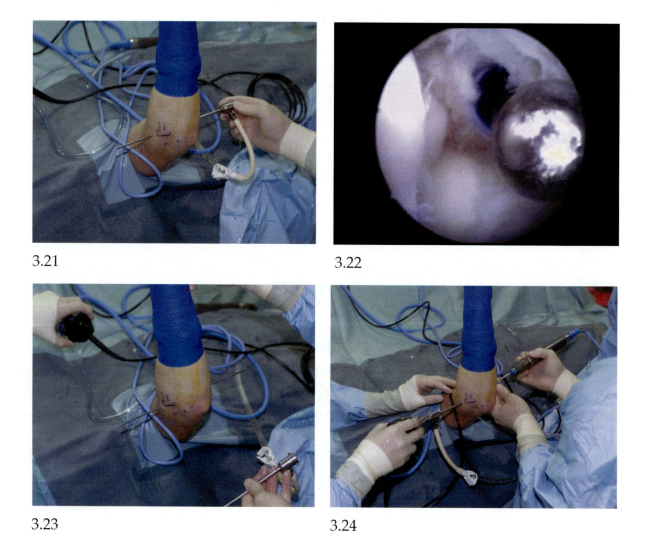

3.21

3.22

3.23

3.24

The posterior aspect of the joint is more difficult to access when the patient is in the supine position, and it is important to have them positioned as far to the edge of the table as possible. It may also be necessary to raise the table and adjust the traction before the portal is created.

Approach the posterior compartment via an incision 1-2 cm proximal to the tip of the olecranon, through the junction between the middle and lateral thirds of the triceps tendon. After a skin incision sharply incise the tendon longitudinally and spread it using a haemostat. The trocar can then be introduced, followed by the arthroscope. This places the arthroscope directly in the olecranon fossa, which is shallow and may provide a very limited view (Fig. 3.25).

Because of the limited space available between the tendon and the posterior humerus it is often easier to create the 'soft spot' portal first, allowing the posterior portal to be fashioned under direct vision. The 'soft spot' portal is made in the same position as the original saline injection site, between the radial head and the olecranon, and is created in the same way as all of the other portals using a skin incision and soft tissue spreading technique (Fig. 3.26).

Once the arthroscope has been introduced via this portal it can be directed back to view the space between the triceps tendon and the posterior aspect of the humerus (Fig. 3.27).

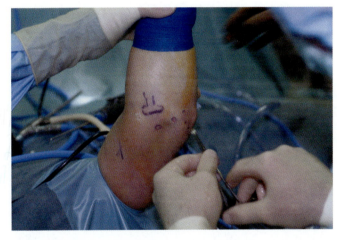

3.25

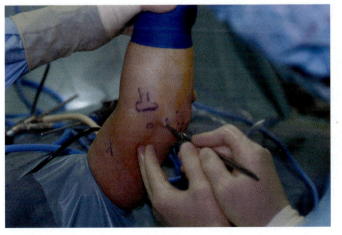

3.26

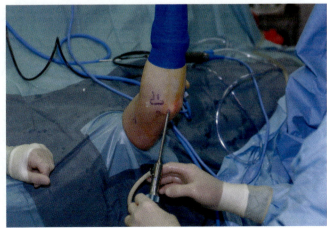

3.27

Make a skin incision for the posterior portal 1–2 cm proximal to the tip of the olecranon and at the junction of the middle and lateral thirds of the tendon (Fig. 3.28).

By introducing a switching stick via this posterior portal the instruments can be switched so that the arthroscope is in the posterior portal, looking back at the soft spot region and the undersurface of the radial head (Fig. 3.29).

Other instruments can then be used via the soft spot portal, which provides better access to the radial head and the joint (Fig. 3.30).

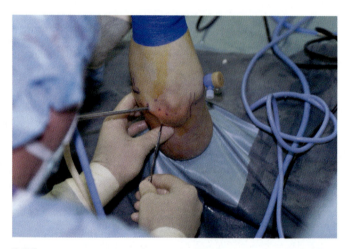

3.28

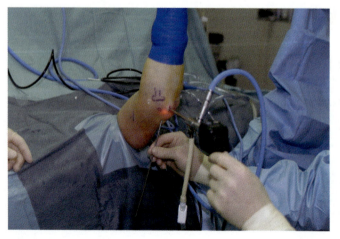

3.29

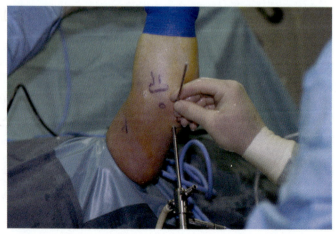

3.30

NORMAL ELBOW ARTHROSCOPY

Prepare and drape the patient as described previously. Create an anteromedial portal as described in the previous section. Use this to guide the creation of an anterolateral portal (Fig. 3.31).

With the arthroscope in the anteromedial portal, identify the radial head. This is used as a landmark for the creation of the anterolateral portal (Fig. 3.32).

Rotate the forearm without flexing or extending the elbow. This will enable the majority of the radial head to be inspected. The portion that cannot be seen via this portal will be seen when the 'soft spot' and posterior portals are created (Fig. 3.33).

The capitellum articulates with the radial head and should be examined next, as this is a common site for chondral fractures producing loose bodies. It is necessary to gently flex and extend the elbow to see the majority of the articular surface. The remainder will be visualized later (Fig. 3.34).

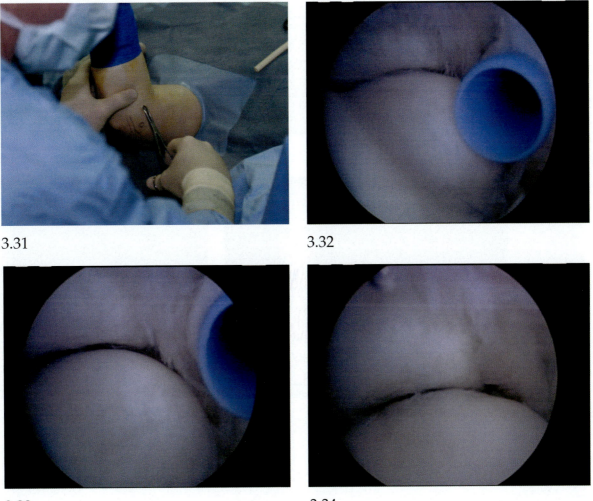

3.31

3.32

3.33

3.34

Inspect the coronoid and the trochlea for osteophytes and impingement. This is often difficult from the medial portal, and often a better view is obtained from the lateral portal (Fig. 3.35).

Inspect the anterior capsule, as this can be released if there is a flexion deformity. In this case there is adequate space and the anterior capsule is not closely adherent (Fig. 3.36).

To examine the medial aspect of the joint it is necessary to switch the instruments, as described previously (Fig 3.37).

Flex the elbow to see the articulation of the coronoid with the trochlea (Fig. 3.38).

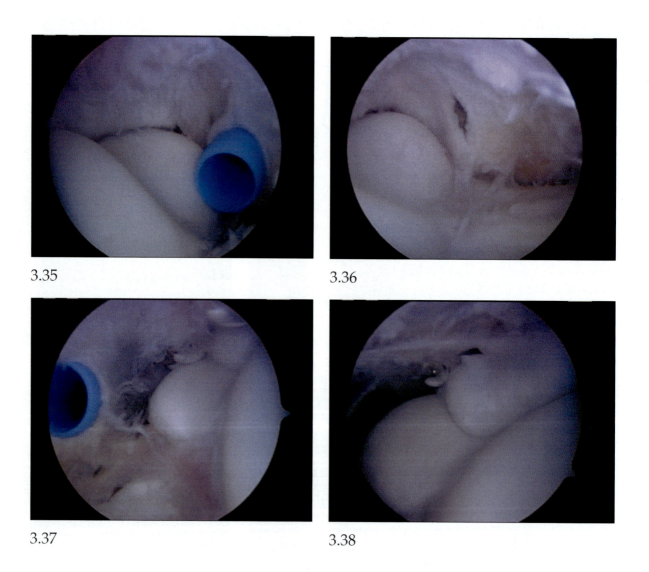

3.35

3.36

3.37

3.38

Extend the elbow and follow the articular surface of the trochlea down anteriorly. This completes the examination of the anterior compartment (Fig. 3.39).

Create the posterolateral 'soft spot' portal as described previously. From here it is possible to view the tip of the olecranon and the olecranon fossa. In this view the horizontal surface is the undersurface of the triceps tendon and the olecranon fossa (Fig. 3.40).

From this portal create the direct posterior portal under direct vision, as described previously, and introduce a switching stick (Fig. 3.41).

By switching the instruments it is then possible to view the lateral gutter. The blue cannula is in the 'soft spot' portal, the olecranon is to the right and the trochlea to the left (Fig. 3.42).

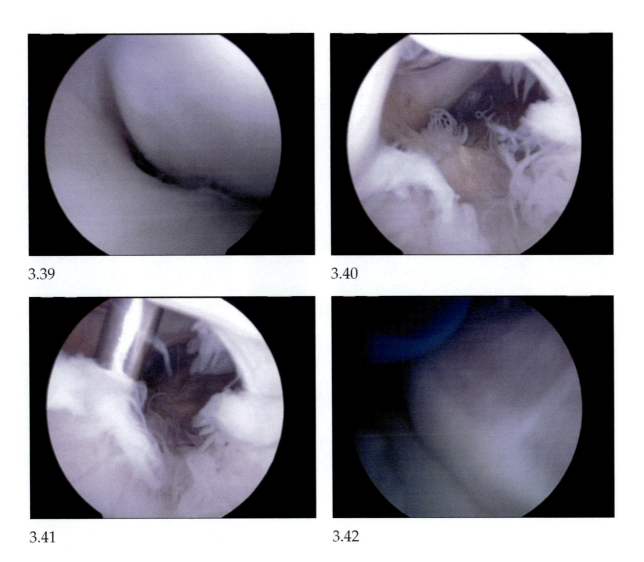

3.39

3.40

3.41

3.42

If the light source is rotated further the inferior aspect of the radial head can be seen. Rotating the forearm enables the examination of this structure to be completed. The radial head is to the left and the ulna to the right (Fig. 3.43).

By carefully advancing and rotating the light source the arthroscope can be manipulated past the lateral aspect of the radial head into a recess. This should be attempted if there is a suspicion of loose bodies, as this is a convenient recess for them to lie in. This area is also difficult to see from either the anteromedial or the anterolateral portals. A loose body can be seen in the centre of this image (Fig. 3.44).

Slowly withdraw the arthroscope. Rotate the light source, and gently flex and extend the elbow to inspect the articulation between the trochlea and the olecranon. There is a consistent area of thinned or absent cartilage on the lateral aspect of the olecranon which should not be confused with pathology. In this image the radial head is seen to the top left of the trochlea ridge inferiorly, and the olecranon and its bare area are to the right (Fig. 3.45).

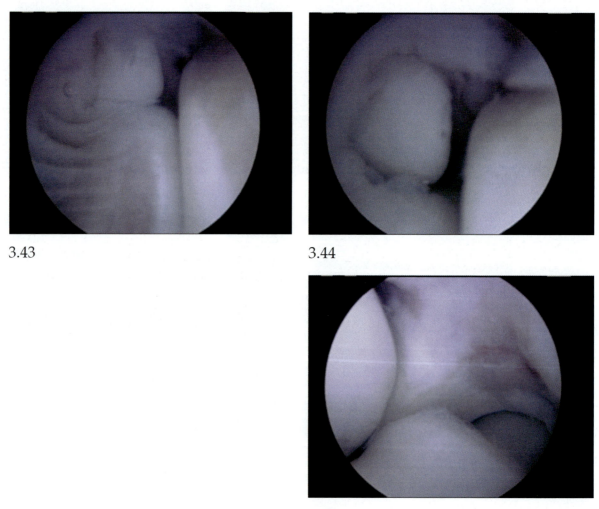

3.43

3.44

3.45

4 WRIST ARTHROSCOPY

INTRODUCTION

Arthroscopy of the wrist is performed far less frequently than of the shoulder or the knee. Specialist instruments are required for this small joint, and arthroscopy should not be attempted without them. The neurovascular and tendinous structures traversing the wrist make careful portal placement essential if damage is to be avoided. Incorrect portal placement also makes both orientation and navigation within the joint difficult. Knowledge of the anatomy is therefore essential. Tension on the musculotendinous unit is required for accurate palpation of the edge of the tendons and subsequent portal placement.

Access to the joint is limited, and a knowledge of the intra-articular anatomy is required.

Only patient setup, portal creation and the normal arthroscopic examination are described in this chapter. More complex procedures are not described and are outside the scope of this book.

There are risks and complications associated with any surgical procedure and the surgeon must be familiar with these before attempting any procedure. The more common or serious ones are outlined here, but there are others which are less common. The surgeon must have knowledge of the applied anatomy of the region if damage is to be avoided.

Neurovascular risks

There are few neurovascular structures at risk in the dorsum of the wrist. Portal 1–2 lies between the terminal branches of the superficial radial nerve and the radial artery. The 6R and 6U portals lie in close proximity to the terminal sensory branches of the ulnar nerve.

The greatest risk is to the tendons, and portal creation which is either made in a sharp fashion or is inaccurate can result in tendon rupture.

162

PATIENT SETUP

The patient is placed supine on the operating table and general anaesthesia is used routinely. If a traction device with a foot plate is to be used (see later) an arm table is required. If weights are to be hung from the upper arm for traction the arm table should be removed. An axillary block may be used as an alternative or to supplement the anaesthesia. A tourniquet is applied above the elbow (Fig. 4.1).

Exsanguinate the hand and forearm using an Eschmark bandage and inflate the tourniquet. The pressure is dependent on the blood pressure and individual preference, but is usually approximately 250 mmHg (Fig. 4.2).

Prepare the hand and arm with iodine down to the elbow. An assistant wearing sterile gloves is required for this (Fig. 4.3).

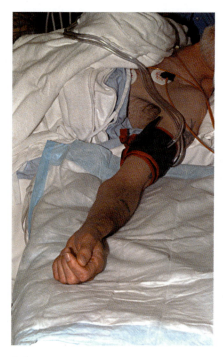 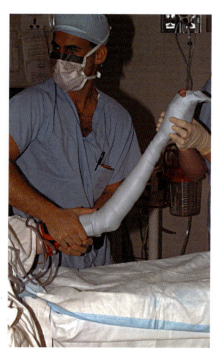 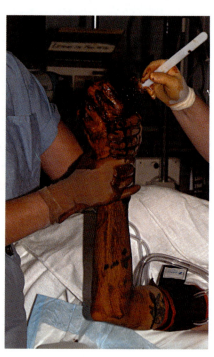

4.1   4.2   4.3

Apply a sterile stockinette and roll it down to the level of the tourniquet. Excess stockinette may have to be removed if it bunches up under the arm (Fig. 4.4).

Apply an extremity drape with a rubber dam over the stockinette, and again bring it above the elbow to the level of the tourniquet (Fig. 4.5).

Cut the stockinette off the hand and wrist and secure the proximal portion with a sterile bandage. Enough stockinette should be removed to leave free access to the wrist and tendons (Fig. 4.6).

There are a number of methods of providing distraction, all using finger traps. The device used in our unit is an integral unit with a foot plate that rests on the arm table. The whole device is sterilized prior to use.

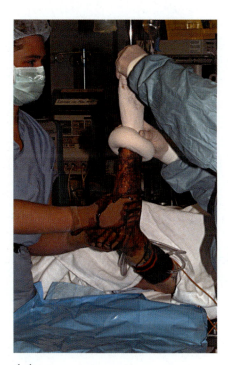

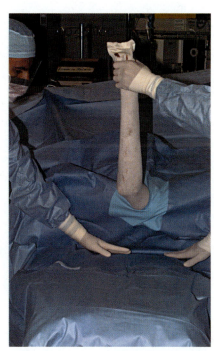

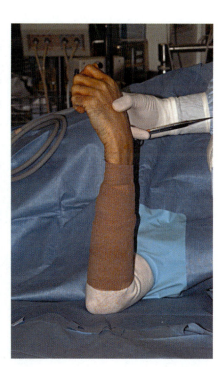

4.4   4.5   4.6

Place the elbow on the foot plate with the palm facing the upright. Wrap the Velcro strap around the forearm. This prevents the arm being lifted up by the traction during the procedure (Fig. 4.7).

Attach the rest of the upright and traction beam to the foot plate (Fig. 4.8).

Apply the finger traps to the index and middle fingers. The ring finger may also be placed in traction if the wrist is being tilted into ulnar deviation (Fig. 4.9).

Hook the beaded chains from the finger traps on to the traction beam. This may necessitate moving the traction beam slightly (Fig. 4.10).

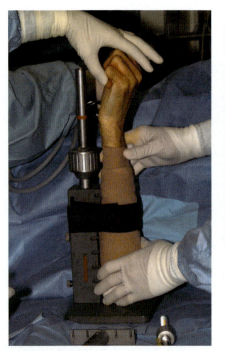

4.7

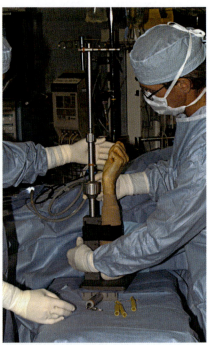

4.8

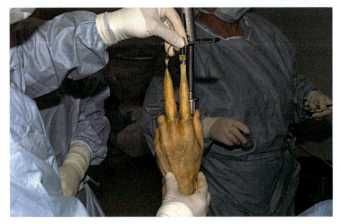

4.9

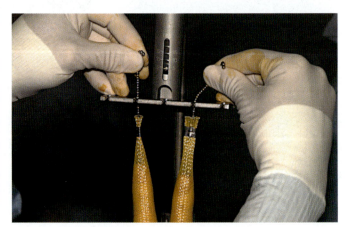

4.10

Adjust the height of the traction beam to produce 5–10 lb traction (Fig. 4.11).

It may be necessary to adjust the traction during the procedure as the arm may migrate upwards despite the Velcro strap. The traction should be checked (Fig. 4.12).

At the completion of setup the traction should appear as in this picture (Fig. 4.13). The forearm is facing the traction upright and, with the finger traps applied, the wrist is not tilted either radial or ulnar.

If this traction device is not available a simpler distraction apparatus can be made by removing the arm table and hanging the fingers by finger traps from a dripstand. 5–10 lb weight is hung from the distal arm, just above the elbow.

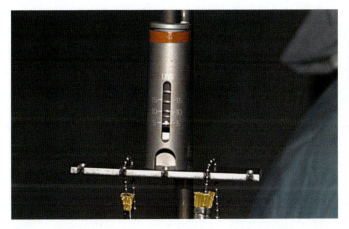

4.11

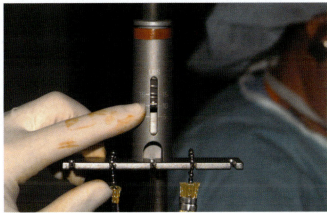

4.12

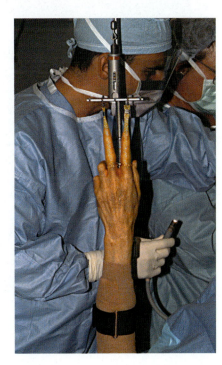

4.13

166

PORTAL PLACEMENT

The patient is placed supine on the operating table and the wrist placed in a distraction device, as described in the previous sections (Fig. 4.13).

Outlining of the landmarks is an essential component of wrist arthroscopy and should be performed before every case. The landmarks not only help in portal placement, but help to keep the surgeon orientated and aware of sites for potential neurovascular damage.

Start by marking the outline of the distal radius and ulna, as well as the level of the carpometacarpal joints. Lister's tubercule can be easily palpated in nearly all patients on the dorsum of the radius, and acts as a landmark for extensor pollicis longus (EPL), which should be indicated. The tendon of extensor digitorum communis (EDC) can be palpated on the ulnar side of this, and should also be drawn (Fig. 4.14).

Palpate the tendon of extensor digitorum minimi (EDM) on the ulnar side of EDC and trace this next (Fig. 4.15).

Extensor carpi radialis brevis (ECRB) can usually be palpated at its insertion, just ulnar to EPL over the carpal bones, and extensor indicis (EI) can often be palpated as it crosses the wrist. If possible, mark both of these. If desired the compartments can be indicated. This is by no means essential, but has been done here for clarity. EPL lies in the third compartment, ECRB in the second and EDC in the fourth (Fig. 4.16).

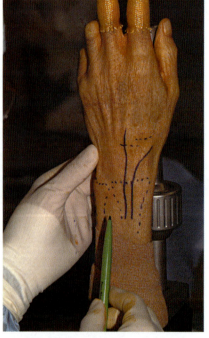 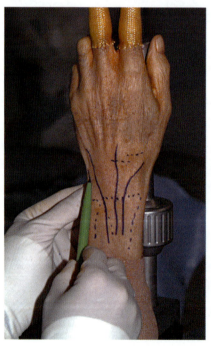 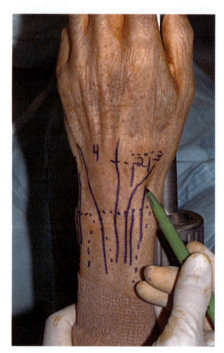

4.14   4.15   4.16

The first portal can now be identified. This is the 3–4 portal and lies between the EPL and the EDC, just above the distal radius. The soft spot can usually be palpated. Mark this spot (Fig. 4.17).

Rotate the wrist slightly and apply a small degree of ulnar deviation. This will enable the extensor carpi ulnaris (ECU) to be palpated lying in the sixth compartment. Draw in the full width of this. Mark a portal on the radial side of this, the '6R' portal (Fig. 4.18).

Mark the '6U' portal on the ulnar side of the tendon (Fig. 4.19).

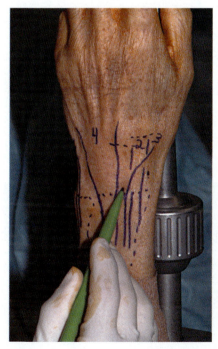

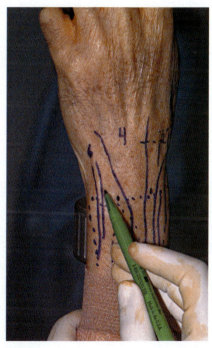

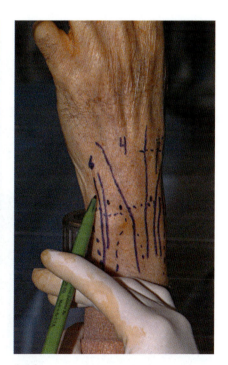

4.17

4.18

4.19

Mark the '4' portal, which splits the tendons of EDC in the midcarpal joint (Fig. 4.20).

The final portal to be marked is the '2–3' portal in the midcarpal joint between the tendons of EPL and EI (Fig. 4.21).

Inflow must be established before an arthroscopic portal can be made. This is done via the 6U portal site. Draw the skin over the tip of the blade to make the incision and blunt dissect with a haemostat down to the capsule (Fig. 4.22).

Insert a small cannula (16–18 g) using a saline-filled syringe. Specific cannulae for wrist arthroscopy are available which have expanded rings along their length to prevent them falling out. If these are not available a simple cannula can be used; however, great care must be taken to prevent them kinking or becoming dislodged (Fig. 4.23).

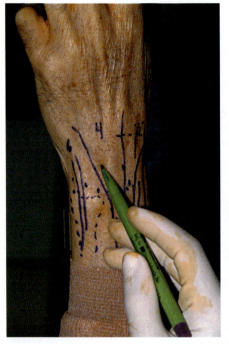
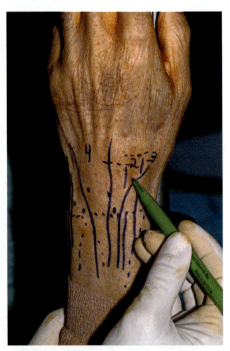

4.20

4.21

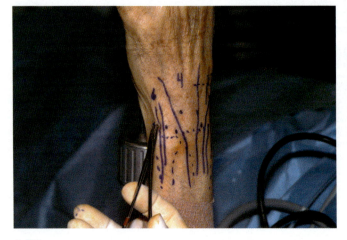
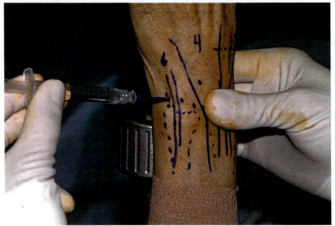

4.22

4.23

Once the tip of the cannula has entered the joint inject 5–10 ml saline. This acts to distend the joint, making subsequent portal placement easier, and also to confirm intra-articular placement of the cannula, as saline will flow back if the syringe is removed and the cannula is in the joint (Fig. 4.24).

Connect the inflow to the cannula once the intra-articular placement has been confirmed. It is advisable to loop the inflow tubing round the little finger to stop it from being dragged out. The first arthroscopic portal can then be made. This is the 3–4 portal, which was previously marked. Again, incise the skin only by drawing the skin over the tip of the knife, and blunt dissect with a haemostat down to the capsule (Fig. 4.25).

Insert the cannula and trocar through the incision into the soft spot. Remember that the radius slopes proximally on the volar side, and aim the trocar accordingly (Fig. 4.26).

As with the inflow cannula, if the trocar is removed and the sleeve is within the joint space saline will flow back out of the cannula (Fig. 4.27).

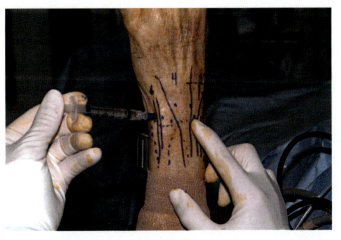

4.24

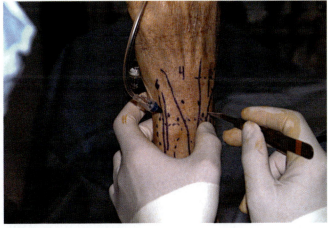

4.25

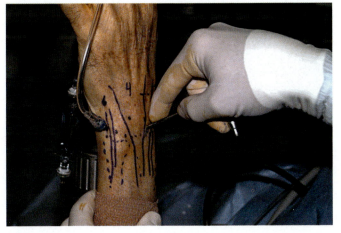

4.26

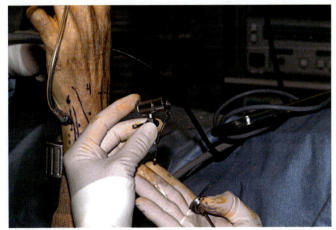

4.27

Once the intra-articular position has been confirmed, insert the arthroscope (Fig. 4.28).

It is recommended that the arthroscope is held in the first web space, balanced between the thumb and index finger. This allows the tip of the middle finger to rest on the skin. If this technique is used it is easy to advance and withdraw the arthroscope and accidental removal is made more difficult (Fig. 4.29).

If the specially designed inflow cannula is used the intra-articular pressure can be increased by squeezing on the small bulb. If this is not used, gentle pressure on the saline bag will achieve the same result (Fig. 4.30).

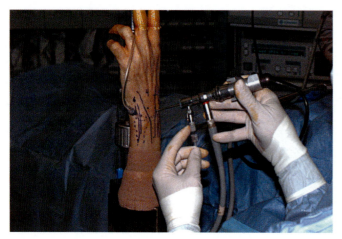

4.28

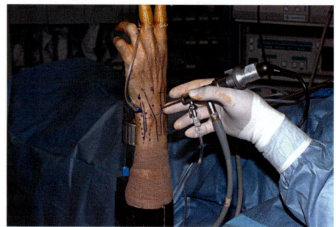

4.29

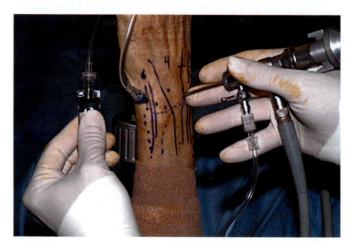

4.30

The first working portal can then be made. Usually this is in the 6R position. Although the approximate position has already been marked, use a spinal needle to confirm that the position is appropriate for any work that may need to be done (Fig. 4.31).

Incise the skin and spread the tissues before any instruments (in this case a shaver) are introduced (Fig. 4.32).

To inspect the midcarpal joints the 4 portal, or EDC-splitting portal, is used. This passes through the tendons of EDC at the midcarpal level (Fig. 4.33).

Again the skin is incised and the soft tissues spread with a haemostat. The blunt trocar is then used to push the tendons aside (Fig. 4.34).

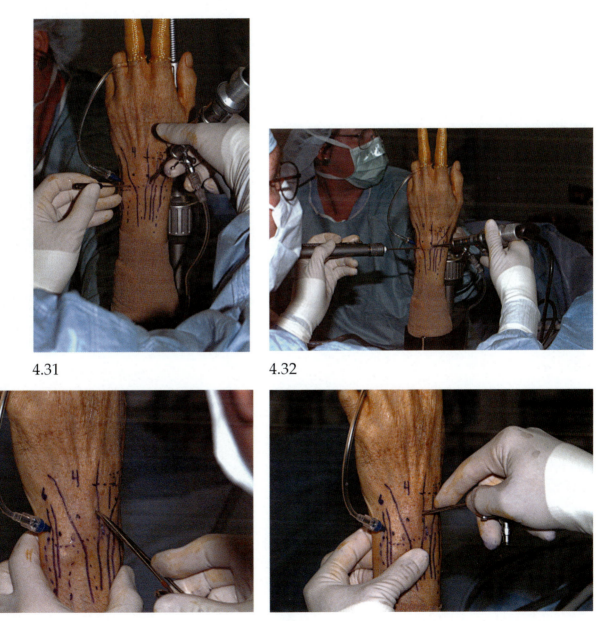

4.31

4.32

4.33

4.34

Once the intra-articular position of the sleeve has been confirmed as before, the arthroscope can be introduced (Fig. 4.35).

Two midcarpal working portals can be made. The first is at the ulnar edge of the EDC tendon and can be located using a spinal needle (Fig. 4.36).

The radial portal is located just above the EPL tendon, in a space created by EPL, ECRB and EI. Again the precise location is identified by a spinal needle, and the incision and blunt dissection procedure follow (Fig. 4.37).

A shaver can be introduced if necessary (Fig. 4.38).

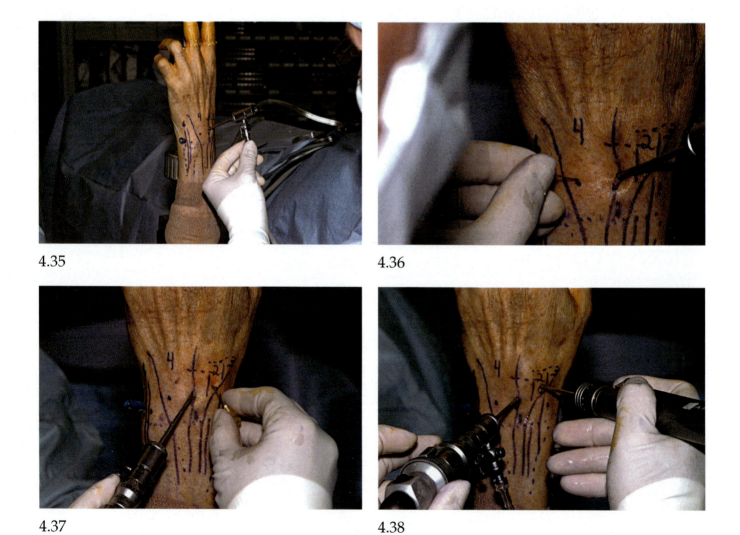

4.35

4.36

4.37

4.38

NORMAL WRIST ARTHROSCOPY

Prepare and drape the patient as described in the previous section.

Insert the inflow cannula into the 6U portal, distend the joint and insert the arthroscope into the 3–4 portal as described. If preferred, a probe can be introduced via the 6R portal, or this can be done at a later stage.

As the arthroscope is introduced into the joint the slightly concave surface of the radius can be seen inferiorly, with the convex scaphoid or lunate above it. What is seen immediately depends on the individual variations in this case the scaphoid is seen to the upper left of the picture (Fig. 4.39).

If the arthroscope is moved gently to the left and right the sagittal ridge, which separates the scaphoid fossa from the lunate fossa, can be identified. There is often slight fraying of this ridge, and this is normal. From here orientation can be achieved. At the volar end of the sagittal ridge a fat pad can be seen consistently. This overlies the radioscapholunate ligament (Fig. 4.40).

Above the sagittal ridge in the normal wrist there is a slight reversal of the convex contour of the scaphoid and the lunate. This is the scapholunate ligament. If it is torn it is possible to drive the arthroscope up into the space, and it may be possible to see the capitate (Fig. 4.41).

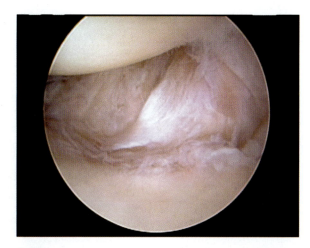

4.39

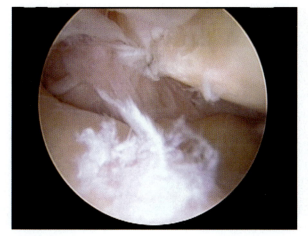

4.40

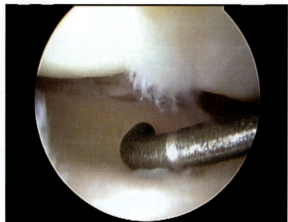

4.41

The scaphoid can then be followed radially and it may be possible to see the triquetrum (Fig. 4.42).

If the arthroscope is then directed to follow the lunate in an ulnar direction, the triangular fibrocartilage can be identified. This will lie underneath the inflow cannula in the 6U portal. The transition between the lunate and the TFCC can best be appreciated with a probe. In this example the TFCC is degenerate, which makes identification easier (Fig. 4.43).

Examination of the midcarpal joints is a routine part of wrist arthroscopy. The arthroscope should be removed from the 3–4 portal and the inflow connected to the arthroscopic sheath.

The preliminary midcarpal portal is the midcarpal radial (MCR) portal. This is located 1 cm distal to the 3–4 portal and is created in the same way as all of the others. The arthroscope is introduced and the inflow turned on when intra-articular placement has been confirmed (Fig. 4.44).

The concavity now seen inferiorly is the scaphoid, and the lunate and the superior convexity is the capitate. A small depression can be seen inferiorly and represents the scapholunate joint (Fig. 4.45).

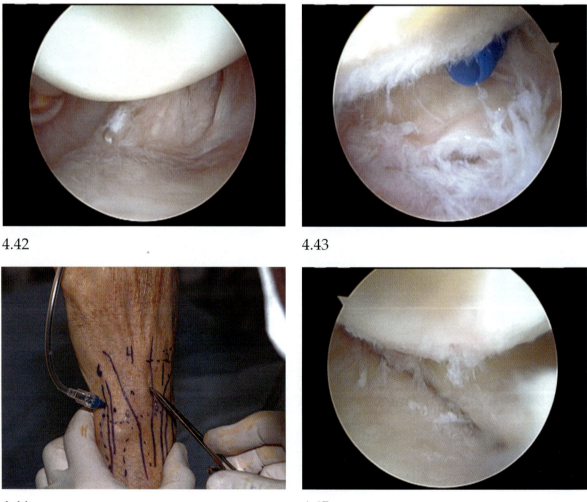

4.42

4.43

4.44

4.45

By rotating the arthroscope radially to follow the capitate (on the right) it is possible to see the trapezoid superiorly, the scaphoid inferiorly (Fig. 4.46).

If the arthroscope is rotated in an ulnar direction the capitate can be seen superiorly, the lunate inferiorly (on the left) and the triquetral on the right. The lunotriquetral joint can also be seen, and if the light source is then rotated superiorly the hamate can be seen (Fig. 4.47).

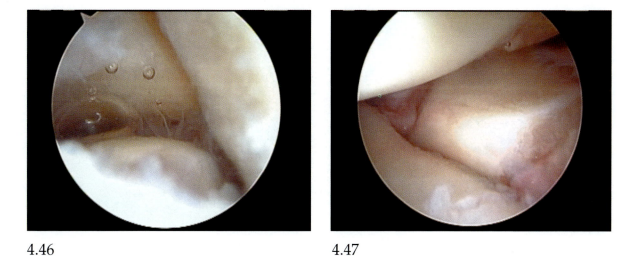

4.46   4.47

5 ANKLE ARTHROSCOPY

INTRODUCTION

Arthroscopy of the ankle, like that of the elbow and wrist, is performed far less frequently than of the shoulder or the knee. The neurovascular and tendinous structures traversing the front, medial aspect and posterior of the ankle make the risk of damage significant if the portals are not placed correctly and carefully.

Access to the joint is limited and care must be taken to avoid chondral damage with the arthroscope.

Only patient setup, portal creation and the normal arthroscopic examination are described in this chapter. Although there are a range of more complex procedures, including debridement and arthrodesis, these are not described and are outside the scope of this book.

There are risks and complications associated with any surgical procedure, and the surgeon must be familiar with these before attempting any procedure. The more common or serious ones are outlined here, but there are others which are less common. The surgeon must have knowledge of the applied anatomy of the region if damage is to be avoided.

Neurovascular risks

The anteromedial portal is positioned close to the long saphenous vein and nerve, whereas the anterocentral portal lies very close to the dorsalis pedis artery, the superficial branch of the deep peroneal nerve, and the medial sensory branch of the superficial peroneal nerve. The lateral sensory branch of the same nerve is in close proximity to the anterolateral portal. The posterocentral portal, through the Achilles tendon, is safe from neurovascular risk. The posterolateral portal puts the sural nerve at risk, particularly if it is made too far from the Achilles tendon. The posterior tibial artery and nerve are jeopardized when the posteromedial portal is used.

PATIENT SETUP

Ankle arthroscopy is generally performed under general anaesthesia. Although regional anaesthesia is an option, however, the patient may find the position uncomfortable.

The patient is placed supine on the operating table and a tourniquet applied to the thigh. The leg is exsanguinated and the tourniquet inflated. A thigh holder of the type used for knee arthroscopy is applied over the tourniquet, and the foot of the table is dropped or removed (Fig. 5.1).

Prepare the leg with iodine to the knee and wrap an impervious U-drape around the thigh, as for a knee arthroscopy (Fig. 5.2).

Roll an impervious stockinette up to the knee and secure it over the leg with a sterile bandage. Place an extremity drape with a rubber dam over the leg (Fig. 5.3).

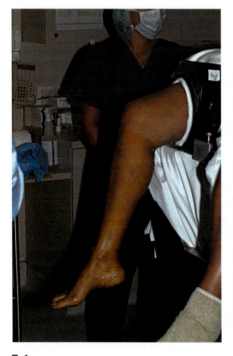

5.1

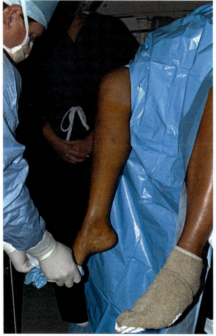

5.2

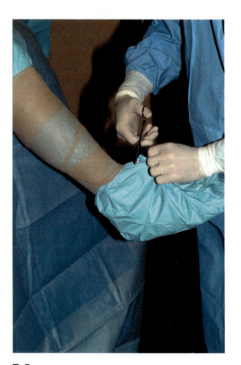

5.3

Cut away the foot portion of the stockinette to expose the ankle (Fig. 5.4).

There are a number of traction devices available for ankle arthroscopy. The simplest is a length of gauze wrapped around the ankle and weighted. This provides good distraction but makes access to the posterior portals difficult. However, in our practice the posterior portals are not used routinely and this is not a problem. Tie 30–40 cm of gauze tape in a loop and wrap it around the ankle as shown. Cross the loop in front of the ankle (Fig. 5.5).

Place the free end of the loop under the foot. Traction on this will allow the ankle to plantar flex (Fig. 5.6).

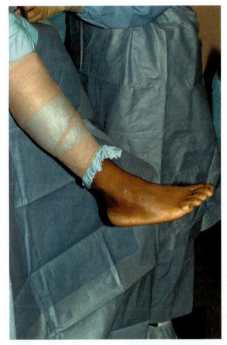

5.4

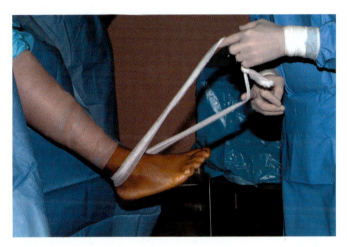

5.5

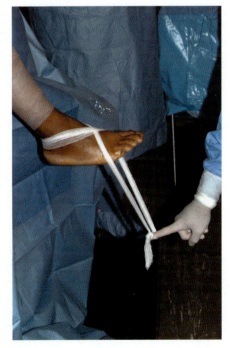

5.6

Weights can then be hung from the loop to provide the traction: 10 lb is usually adequate (Fig. 5.7).

To prevent the gauze from chafing the foot, wrap a length of sterile bandage under the loop (Fig. 5.8).

To prevent the tape from slipping during the procedure, secure it to the foot with bandage (Fig. 5.9).

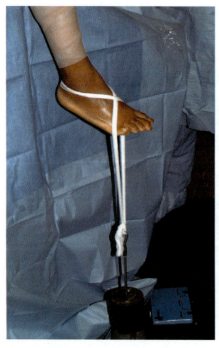

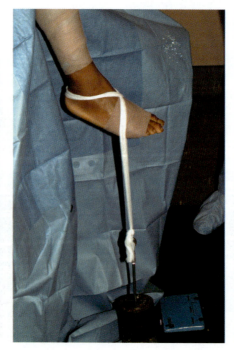

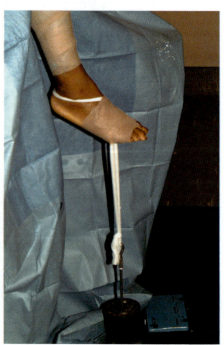

5.7   5.8   5.9

PORTAL PLACEMENT

The patient is set up on the operating table as described in the previous section, and traction is applied to the foot.

Draw the anatomical landmarks on the anterior ankle. Draw the tibiotalar joint as a horizontal line. Draw the tibialis anterior tendon medially and the lateral edge of extensor digitorum minimi (EDM) laterally. Draw the anterior edge of the fibula also, as this defines the area for the lateral portal. Outline the medial border of extensor digitorum communis (EDC), as this provides a landmark for the dorsalis pedis artery (Fig. 5.10).

A number of portals have been described. We do not routinely use posterior portals, as the risk of damage to neurovascular structures is high and the benefit gained is low. The anterocentral portal, which splits the EDC tendon, is also not used because of the risk of damaging the dorsalis pedis artery.

The anteromedial portal is the initial arthroscopic portal used routinely. It is located at the level of the joint line medial to the medial edge of tibialis anterior. In this region there is a risk of damaging the saphenous nerve and vein, and so care must be taken (Fig. 5.11).

Identify the portal site and inject 10–15 ml saline into the joint via this portal. The soft spot between the lateral edge of EDM and the fibula will be seen to bulge as the ankle fills with fluid. The insertion of the needle will also confirm the level of the joint in relation to the proposed portal site (Fig. 5.12).

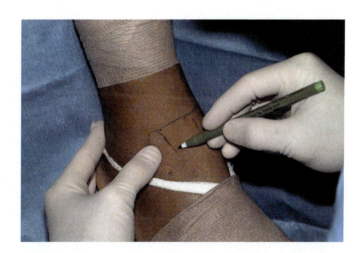

5.10

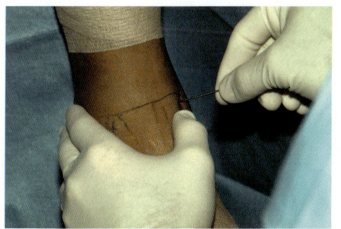

5.11

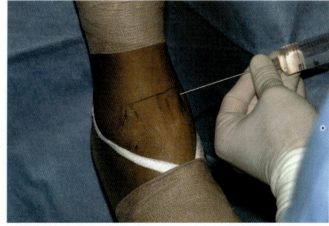

5.12

Make a skin incision for the anteromedial portal by drawing the skin over the tip of a number 11 blade. Do not push the blade through the skin. This incision technique should be used for the creation of all the portals around the ankle, wrist and elbow, to avoid damaging the nerves when they are subcutaneous in these areas (Fig. 5.13).

Use a short blunt trocar and sleeve to push through the capsule. Aim the trocar at the front of the tibia. Allow it to run across laterally as the joint is entered. If the trocar is removed the saline will flow back if the sleeve is within the joint (Fig. 5.14).

The arthroscope can then be introduced. A standard 4.5 mm 30° arthroscope is preferred as this gives a larger field of view and is familiar to all arthroscopic surgeons. A small joint arthroscope can be used, although it can be difficult to see enough of the joint at any one time (Fig. 5.15).

The lateral, working portal can then be created. This is done under direct vision. The site for the lateral portal is the soft spot between the lateral edge of EDM and the anterior edge of the fibula. Confirm the correct position with an 18 g spinal needle. Once the needle is seen within the joint, confirm that all areas can be reached from that position (Fig. 5.16).

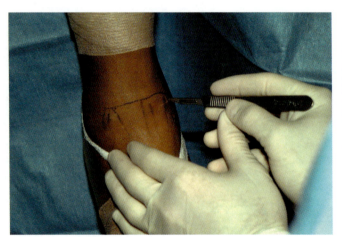

5.13

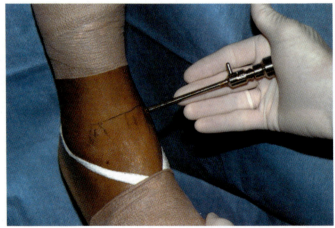

5.14

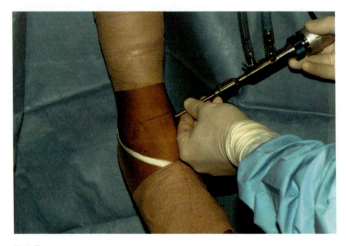

5.15

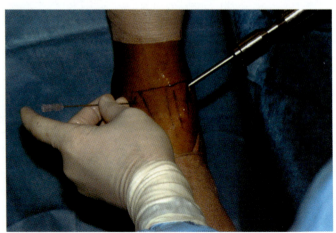

5.16

Incise the skin as previously described and use a haemostat to blunt dissect down to the capsule (Fig. 5.17).

Insert a short blunt trocar as described previously, aiming across the front of the joint to reduce the risk of chondral damage. This is guided by direct vision (Fig. 5.18).

Alternatively, a short blue 4.5 mm cannula can be used. This has the advantages of providing a more secure purchase on the soft tissues, reducing the risk of losing the portal and reducing the risk of chondral damage. A probe or other instrument can then be introduced via this portal (Fig. 5.19).

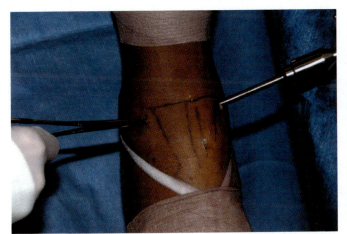

5.17

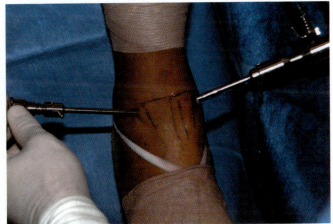

5.18

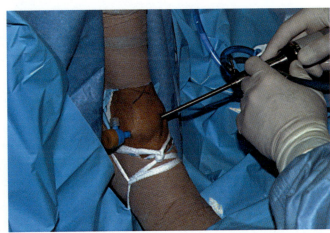

5.19

NORMAL ANKLE ARTHROSCOPY

The patient is prepared and draped as described previously (Fig. 5.20).

Outline the anatomical landmarks and create the anteromedial and anterolateral portals created, as described previously (Fig. 5.21).

With the arthroscope in the anteromedial portal the examination begins in the medial gutter. Here the deep portion of the deltoid ligament and the medial gutter can be seen.

By rotating the light source the medial talar dome can be seen (Fig. 5.22).

Bring the arthroscope out of the medial gutter and laterally across the joint. The medial talar articulation with the tibial plafond can be seen, as well as the sagittal groove (Fig. 5.23).

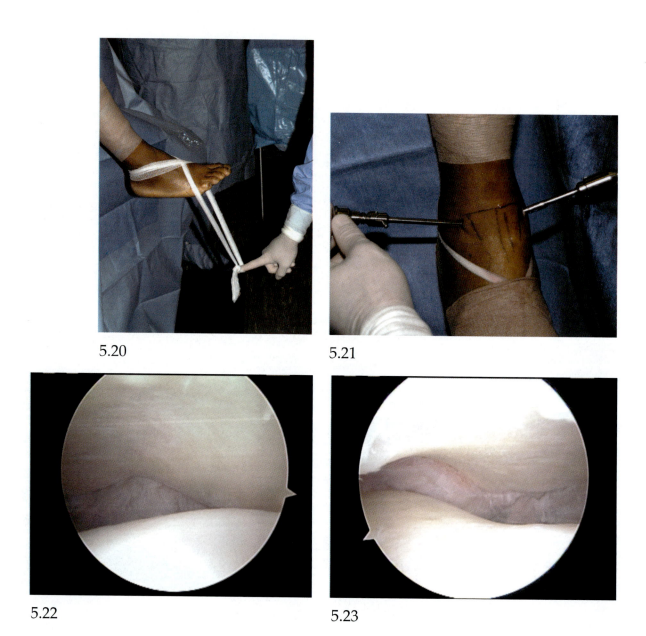

5.20

5.21

5.22

5.23

The medial dome of the talus and articular surface of the corresponding tibia can then be viewed. At this stage it may be possible to see the capsular reflection of flexor hallucis longus by advancing the arthroscope towards the posteromedial wall (Fig. 5.24).

Withdraw the arthroscope slightly to continue the inspection of the major articular surfaces (Fig. 5.25).

Move the arthroscope towards the lateral gutter. Here the gutter itself can be visualized, as well as the distal fibular articulation with the talus. The posterior inferior tibiofibular ligament and the transverse tibiofibular ligament can also be seen from this position (Fig. 5.26).

Draw the arthroscope anteriorly to inspect the anterior gutter from lateral to medial (Fig. 5.27).

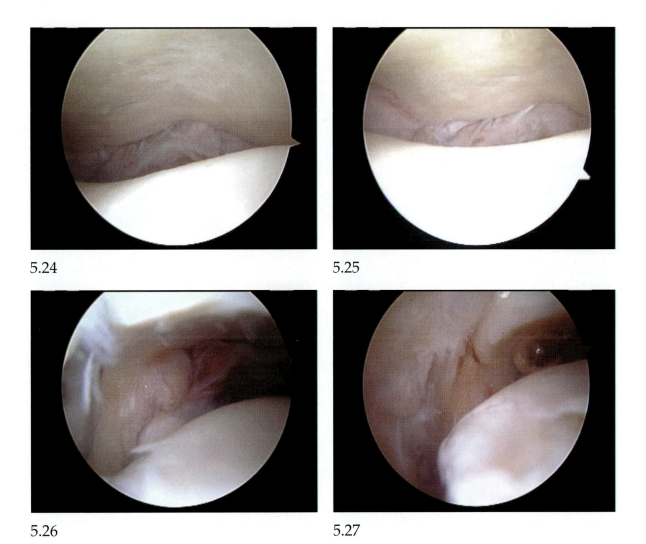

5.24

5.25

5.26

5.27

INDEX